**Geoffrey Cannon** read iology at Balliol College of *New Society* magazine, and editor of *Radio Times* from 1969–1979. But he only started to enjoy himself when he stopped cutting calories in the late 1970s. In 1983 he wrote *Dieting Makes You Fat*, with Hetty Einzig. This first book was a best-seller in Britain, America, Canada, Australia and Europe.

*The Food Scandal*, written with Caroline Walker in 1984, was another immediate bestseller. It showed why the British food supply, heavy in unhealthy fats, sugars and additives, makes us ill, and fat too.

In 1983, he discovered that the expert NACNE report on dietary goals for Britain had been suppressed by Government for over two years. As a result, he wrote the *Sunday Times* features that first revealed the existence of that report. He has also written major articles on food and health for the *Observer* and *The Times*. He writes regularly for *New Health* magazine, of which he is Consultant Editor.

From 1980 to 1984 he was an Assistant Editor at *The Sunday Times*. In 1985 he was named Best Specialist Columnist in the Magazine Publishing Awards.

He has written the 'Fun Runner' column for *Running* magazine since 1980, and started *The Sunday Times* 'Getting in Shape' project in 1983. He is a director of London Road Runners Club, and can occasionally be seen running, slowly, round Hyde Park.

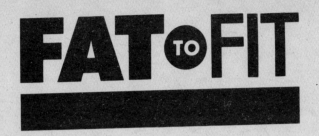

# FAT TO FIT

## Geoffrey Cannon

**A PAN ORIGINAL**

**PAN BOOKS LONDON AND SYDNEY**

First published 1986 by Pan Books Ltd,
Cavaye Place, London SW10 9PG
9 8 7 6 5 4 3 2 1
© Fat to Fit text, Geoffrey Cannon 1986
Wheel of Health name and device are registered trade marks,
© Geoffrey Cannon and Caroline Walker. Reproduction
forbidden without written permission.
Recipe for Leek and Ham Sauce (p.161) reproduced from
*The Taste of Health* edited by Jenny Rogers, with the permission
of the British Broadcasting Corporation.
ISBN 0 330 29614 0
Photoset by Parker Typesetting Service, Leicester
Printed and bound in Great Britain by
Cox & Wyman Ltd, Reading

# A PROMISE
# AND A CAUTION

There are no false promises of quick, permanent weight loss in FAT TO FIT. If you have ever gone on a calorie-cutting campaign, you will know that you lose weight at first. What you may not know is that little of this initial weight loss is of body fat and, as a rule, as soon as the calorie-cutting ends, the weight – and the fat – goes back on again. Sounds familiar?

A caution. If you are very fat (more than thirty pounds overweight, say), or if you really do eat or drink a lot more than other people, or can't stop yourself gorging, look for professional support. Following the FAT TO FIT plan, or trying to, can't do you any harm and can only do you good. It's all about healthy eating, together with a healthy amount of activity that every able-bodied person can fit in, every day. But FAT TO FIT will not magic your fat, or your problems, away.

If you have picked up FAT TO FIT because you are reasonably healthy but haven't found the way to budge those bulges, then this is the book and the plan for you. Over six months you will feel good, lose fat, and become slimmer. And that's a promise.

For Caroline

For more than one reason what I publish here will have points of contact with what other people are writing today. If my remarks do not bear a stamp which marks them as mine, I do not wish to lay any further claim to them as my property.

Ludwig Wittgenstein
Philosophical Investigations

# ACKNOWLEDGEMENTS

Science is, or should be, nothing more than knowledge and ideas brought together for the common good. Highly trained specialists who keep their work secret fail as citizens and as scientists. Societies are moved only by ideas that everybody can understand. Many generous people have encouraged me to collate their research and to find a pattern in it. Above all I owe special thanks to Dr Denis Burkitt, Professor Michael Crawford, Dr Kenneth Heaton, Professor Philip James, Dr Hugh Sinclair, Dr Hugh Trowell, Caroline Walker, and Professor Arvid Wretlind. The responsibility for this book is mine. Much of the credit is theirs.

A team of people made the book. The designer is Robin Allen, the publisher (at Pan) Hilary Davies, the editor Carl Gardner, the secretary Carole Hobson. Adriana Luba turned the meals into Wheels, Wendy Doyle checked them, Roger Phillips took the colour photographs and John Ireland drew the jokes. Deirdre McQuillan and Adriana Luba devised the weekly plans starting on page 155. Eric Verdon-Roe said to keep it simple and Caroline Walker looked at the facts.

While the book and the judgements in it are mine, more thanks for guidance in its preparation or for supply of information go to Professor Per-Olof Åstrand, Professor Norman Blacklock, Professor Derek Bryce-Smith, Dr David Buss, Professor John Catford, Dr David Cummings, Professor John Durnin, Dr John Garrow, Dr Paula Geiselman, Dr Walter Hare, Professor William Haskell, Professor Mark Hegsted, Dorothy Hollingsworth, Dr David Horrobin, Dr Michael Jacobson, Sir Francis Avery Jones, Dr Tim Lang, Professor Barry Lewis, Dr Alan Long, Alistair Mackie, Professor Thomas McKeown, Dr Donald McLaren, Melanie Miller, Dr Erik Millstone, Professor Jerry Morris, Dr Eric Newholme, Professor Ralph Paffenbarger, Dr Andrew Prentice, Dr Sheldon Reiser, Margaret Sanderson, Professor Aubrey Sheiham, Professor John Soothill, Dr David Southgate, Professor Jeremiah

Stamler, Professor Stewart Truswell, Colin Tudge, Professor Mark Wahlqvist, Dr Werner Wheelock, Dr Roger Williams, Professor Peter Wood, Arthur Wynn, Margaret Wynn, Dr Walter Yellowlees and Professor John Yudkin.

I also owe thanks to Magnus Linklater and Nicholas Wapshott of *The Observer*; to Mike Cheyne, Gary Day-Ellison, Jacqueline Graham, Margaret Heriot and Sonny Mehta at Pan; to Mike Baldwin, Carole Handslip and Alex Henderson; and, as always, to Deborah Rogers.

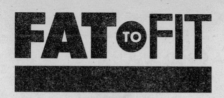

# CONTENTS

# FAT TO FIT

## ALL YOU NEED TO KNOW

**H**ere's how to lose your excess fat forever, while keeping your friends, family, health and sanity ● Dieters have been trained to fear food and to go hungry all the time. But calorie-cutting diets don't work ● For good health everybody needs lots of whole, fresh food ● And here is the best possible news for slimmers: if you enjoy your fill of healthy food, and restore some everyday action into your life, you will gain energy and lose fat. FAT TO FIT is the plan to use for transforming the quality of your life

'It doesn't make any difference what I eat' people so often say. 'I still get fat.' If this is what you feel, FAT TO FIT is news. For the fact is that what you eat makes all the difference between being fat and being slim.

'You can't eat anything nowadays' people are beginning to say. 'Everything is bad for you.' If this is what you are beginning to think, FAT TO FIT is good news. For what you eat makes all the difference between being unhealthy and being healthy.

'It's all so confusing' everybody is saying. 'I can't cope

with all these new stories about food and health.' If this is what you say, FAT TO FIT is better news. For the food you need for energy and positive health, and the food you need to protect you against all sorts of diseases, *is the same food* you need to make and keep you slim.

The best news of all is that the only reliable way to lose your extra fat for ever is to enjoy your fill of delicious, nourishing food. Yes, it's true. FAT TO FIT is the first book to show why and how you can move from Fat to Fit, starting today.

The problem with the British food supply today is not too much quantity, but not enough quality. We eat less than our grandparents, but are fatter. Compared with a couple of generations ago, it's been calculated that we eat a tenth less and weigh a tenth more. So forget about the starvation and malnutrition of calorie-cutting. Hunger is not just for calories (energy) but also for nourishment.

In common with other Western countries, the British food supply is heavy in saturated fats and added sugars, made palatable in highly processed food by the sophisticated use of chemical additives. Processed, concentrated food is least satisfying, and most likely to make you fat and leave you hungry. One reason is that it simply doesn't fill you up. Another is that highly processed food is so drained of nourishment that it deprives your body. The only way to get enough nourishment from highly processed food is to eat excess calories. It is literally true that sedentary people who eat typical British food now, have the choice of getting ill or getting fat – or fat and ill.

You don't believe it? Well, here's an interesting fact. The food manufactured for domestic, farm, zoo and laboratory animals is much more nourishing than food manufactured for humans. If you feed your dog with human food it will become listless, depressed and constipated; it will be likely to suffer, and die prematurely from heart disease or cancer, and it will get fat. We are no different. The food on offer nowadays is not fit for a dog, cow, ape or rat.

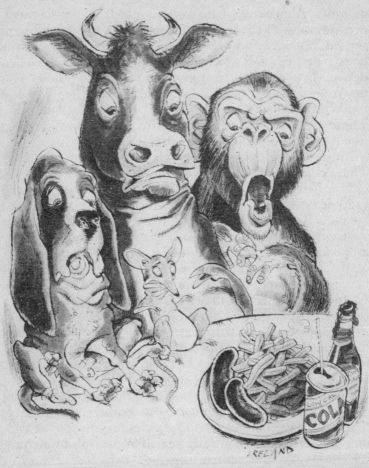

Dieters have been trained to fear food and to go hungry all the time. But if you choose the right food, always preferring food that's whole and fresh, big hearty meals are a vital part of the plan to lose body fat. Diet books claim or imply that the basic requirement of our bodies is for energy (measured as calories) and that all we need to do to lose fat is cut calories. The diet books are wrong.

First, the body's requirement is for quality, not just

17

quantity. Above all, what the body needs is nourishment. Second, most of the weight lost on a calorie-cutting diet is not fat, but water and lean tissue, including glycogen, the body's immediately available energy store which, when depleted, makes you hungry. Third, dieting slows you down and trains the body to make do with less and less food, thus causing the condition it is supposed to cure. These are some of the reasons why *Dieting Makes You Fat* (the title of a book I co-wrote with Hetty Einzig).

But if dieting does make you fat, what makes you slim? That's what FAT TO FIT is all about.

The bad news about the food supply is shown in the graphic device shown opposite, which I call 'The Wheel of Health'. This is a map of nourishment. It is a way of showing the quality of a food, a meal, or the diet of an individual or a nation, at a glance. The Wheel opposite is empty; it shows what almost half of our food supply looks like: totally empty of nourishment, devoid of satisfaction. A 'full' Wheel, with all its segments filled in, shows a properly balanced and varied diet. Throughout FAT TO FIT, I show you how you can transform the quality of your food, meal by meal, day by day, for the six months or so it takes to move from Fat to Fit. You will gain energy and health, while losing fat and eating your fill.

People in Britain today get fat not just because machine-made concentrated food leaves us empty and hungry. Machines have turned us into a sedentary people, travelling by car, living in centrally heated houses, and watching television. We are trained to prefer convenience, and to avoid any kind of physical activity. We are discouraged from making an effort.

And tiny differences – pre-sliced bread, electric type-writers, automatic gear-shifts – between our way of life and that of our grandparents, accumulate. 'Labour-saving' means that our bodies are able to use less and less energy. In scientific language, the 'energy balance' of people in Britain and other Western countries is dropping lower

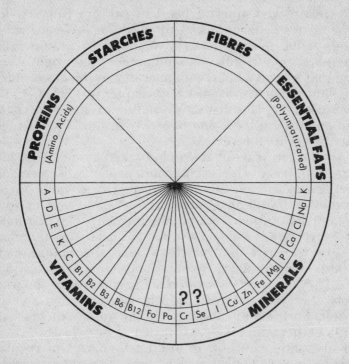

**● Sweet fat Wheel of Health: saturated fats and processed sugars.**
The Wheel of Health is a map of nourishment. A full wheel shows a
balanced diet. Two-thirds of our food supply is fats, sugars and
alcohol. This empty wheel is of saturated fats and processed sugars:
totally empty of nourishment, they make us ill ... and fat, too.
(Detailed explanation of the Wheel: page 181.)

and lower. But while we get fat on less and less calories,
our body's need for nourishment stays the same.

The way that modern nutritionists explain this crisis,
which makes us unfit, unhealthy, and fat, is that what we
need is 'nutrient-dense' food; but what we're getting is
'calorie-dense' food. In plain language this means that the
way to move from Fat to Fit is to transform the quality of
the food you eat. You can do this by making new choices in

any well-stocked supermarket. Fit food isn't 'funny' food. As a matter of fact, a lot of the traditional Great British food eaten by previous generations is healthy and slimming. Quite often grandmother was right. For example, a good way for a slimmer to start the day is with a big, hot, filling breakfast. Every chapter of FAT TO FIT gives detailed plans that show you how to choose, prepare and enjoy good food, and how easy it is to kick Fat food out of your life forever.

After some years of research, backed by meetings and correspondence with leading independent doctors and scientists in Britain, Europe and America, some featured here, I've found that modern knowledge and ancient wisdom about food are now in agreement. The best food for everybody is whole, fresh food. That's what the fibre experts are saying. And that's what the independent experts on fats, sugars, vitamins and minerals are saying, too. They are specialists, often not in communication with each other, often using abstract language of no use to lay people. FAT TO FIT has brought the work of these scientists together and, I hope, expressed it more clearly.

I also show you how to lose fat by means of regular activity any able-bodied person can make part of everyday life. The way to a new slim you isn't only by lots of vigorous exercise. People who exercise a lot are in any case likely to be fit and slim already. FAT TO FIT is about everyday choices. It shows you how to choose and pick good food, and how to recover your lost energy.

FAT TO FIT is a guide. It's also a game that everybody can play, with something to look at and check out on every page. It's for slimmers and for everybody else too. You need never slim alone again. Plenty of good food and plenty of fresh air is the best way of life for everybody. Enjoy FAT TO FIT, and enjoy yourself, your family and your friends.

Geoffrey Cannon
London 1986

# FAT TO FIT

## 1

# MOVEABLE FEASTS

**We have more choices of food than ever before. Three set meals are a thing of the past. Anybody who lives in a town can go down the road and pick up a quick lunch from a sandwich bar ● But what's a good choice? Here's how to tell the difference between a lunch that will make you Fat, and a lunch that will make you Fit ● All about bread that's Fit to eat ● And there's more good news: the right food for slimmers fills you up and leaves you satisfied, not hungry ● Plus, why you can say goodbye forever to the misery and failures of yo-yo dieting**

Everybody eats sandwich lunches. Kids take them to school; office workers take them away from sandwich bars; they're quick and easy to make up at home. Portable lunches should be delicious, filling, satisfying – and a vital part of the FAT TO FIT plan.

Both the lunches analysed on pages 24–25 and pictured on pages 98–99 contain around 700 calories of energy, including the snack that might be kept for the afternoon. This is roughly one third of the energy an average-sized woman needs every day.

The most obvious immediate difference between the

two meals is their size. The fattening meal takes up a small space, on the counter and in your stomach. This is because much of it is highly concentrated calories: fats in the bacon and margarine (or butter), and in the crisps; fats and sugars in the confectionery.

People who try to be careful about their weight (meaning, fat), without actually going on a calorie-cutting campaign, often try to compensate for something tasty but obviously fatty, like a bacon sandwich, by restricting themselves to nibbles like crisps for the rest of the meal, together with painless 'slimmers' items like soft drinks containing chemical sweeteners. The trouble is, though, that a meal like this, as well as being decidedly unhealthy, is liable to leave you hungry. Hence the small bar of confectionery, which will probably set you up for another nibble, like a couple of sweet biscuits with afternoon tea.

It's hard to believe that two sandwiches are better than one if you want to lose fat, partly because dieting books have often claimed (wrongly) that bread is fattening, and partly because the healthy meal shown on page 99 is bulky, and therefore filling and satisfying. Common sense might suggest that the way to lose fat is to eat food that leaves you feeling hungry. In this case, on the whole, common sense is wrong. Tasty sandwich fillings like tuna or banana will fill you up and are less likely to lead to mid-afternoon cravings for sweetened things.

Two sandwiches with healthy fillings supply more calories than one sandwich with a fatty filling. But the Fit meal also adds up to 700 calories, because plain yoghurt and whole fruit are light in calories and rich in nourishment, whereas crisps and confectionery are heavy in calories but drained of nourishment.

So that you can see the difference between Fat and Fit food there are menus (see opposite) and Wheels of Health for Fat and Fit meals (see pages 24, 25 and 27) here and throughout the book.

Bacon is a very fattening filling. Any concentrated pro-

# THE CHOICE IS YOURS

**SANDWICH BAR LUNCH**
(photographs: pages 98, 99)

| | FAT<br>700 calories | FIT (1)<br>700 calories | FIT (2)<br>700 calories |
|---|---|---|---|
| | Bacon sandwich (white bread) Crisps No-cal drink | Tuna sandwich (wholemeal bread) Banana sandwich (wholemeal bread) Plain yoghurt (6 oz) | Sardines (3½ oz) Potato salad (3½ oz) Mixed salad: butter beans (3½ oz), tomatoes (4 oz), celery (2 oz), mushroom (2 oz), parsley, French dressing (1 scant tbsp), wholemeal roll (large) |
| | Confectionery (small item) | Apple Orange | Peach 2 Apricots |
| Saturated fats | HEAVY | LIGHT | LIGHT |
| Sugars | MEDIUM | LIGHT | LIGHT |
| Salt | HEAVY | MEDIUM | MEDIUM |
| Additives | HEAVY | LIGHT | LIGHT |
| Proteins | RICH | SUPER-RICH | SUPER-RICH |
| Starches | POOR | MEDIUM | RICH |
| Fibres | POOR | SUPER-RICH | SUPER-RICH |
| Essential fats | POOR | RICH | SUPER-RICH |
| Vitamin C | POOR | SUPER-RICH | SUPER-RICH |
| Folic acid (Fo) | POOR | RICH | RICH |
| Potassium (K) | POOR | RICH | SUPER-RICH |
| Zinc (Zn) | POOR | MEDIUM | RICH |

Key to terms used here and on Wheels of Health: page 199.
Sandwich and salad recipes: Chapter 9.

cessed fats or sugars, such as sausage, pâté, salami, cheese and pickle, or jam, are fattening; the more so with margarine or butter added. By contrast, nourishing and satisfying fillings add protein to starchy wholemeal bread, without saturated fats or added sugars. If you don't fancy tuna or other fish, poultry or lean meat is a good choice.

There aren't many sweet whole foods like banana that

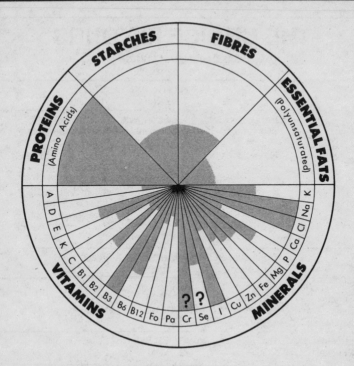

● **Fat sandwich bar lunch: bacon and processed snacks.** The bacon, like any meat, supplies proteins, but this lunch is a disaster. It's fatty, sugary and salty, and loaded with additives. The fats and sugars drive out the nourishing vitamins and minerals. What's worse, its 700 calories won't satisfy you. No-cal drinks are chemicals and emptiness. White bread will bung you up. (Photograph: page 98. Menu: page 23).

work as sandwich fillings, so if you don't fancy two fish or meat sandwiches, or if you are vegetarian, home-made soups made from fresh vegetables (and no added salt!), and baked potatoes, are excellent choices. Avoid fatty garnishes and, instead, add lots of lemon (not margarine) to the tuna, and tangy onion slices with a bit of cheese (not butter) to the baked potato.

Be fussy. Look for a sandwich bar where the choice of

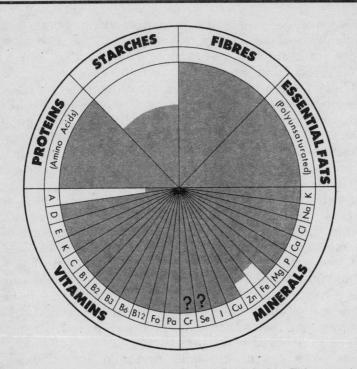

● **Fit sandwich bar lunch: wholemeal and fruits.** This contains exactly the same 700 calories as the Fat lunch opposite, but it's packed with nourishment. The Wheel is almost completely full, showing a balanced meal. More good news is that this meal will fill you up. You can save the fruit for a snack: fruit's natural sweetness comes with fibres, vitamins and minerals. (Photograph: page 99. Menu: page 23. Recipe: page 174.)

delicatessen, vegetables and salads is good. Praise traders who like to make up sandwiches to your specification, who will use lemon rather than oil, who prefer substantial wholemeal bread, who make their own soups.

Eat as many vegetables and fruits as you like, with any meal or between meals, but don't substitute salads for filling whole starchy food.

Some foods, like red meat, cheese and eggs, are 'in-between' choices as sandwich fillings; all right once in a while or for a change, but not every day. Cheese of most types, for example, is rather more a high-fat than a high-protein food, and best used as a garnish.

Other foods with a supposedly healthy image, such as granola or muesli bars, 'raw sugar' bars, exotic items like halva, or dried fruit and nuts, are nourishing, but nevertheless are concentrated calories. On the other hand, some whole foods rejected as high calorie by the diet books, such as avocados and fatty fish, are exceedingly nourishing and satisfying.

Sandwiches are ingenious packages of food, handy as part of a take-away meal, a packed school lunch or for a picnic. But just how nourishing a sandwich is depends, of course, on the quality of the bread and what's inside.

Sliced, white bread, that damp, chemicalized fluff, will bung you up and do you no good. When Alistair Mackie was director general of the Health Education Council, he made himself unpopular with the British millers and bakers by saying that, as far as he could see, the only sensible use of pre-packed white bread was as a filler for mouse-holes or cracks in the wall. And nobody eats mass-produced white bread by itself. It's disgusting! This is why sandwiches have got a bad reputation, most of all among slimmers. The only way to make white bread palatable is to fill it with strong-tasting salty and/or fatty items, such as bacon, or else spread it with fats (butter or margarine), and sugary products such as jam and marmalade. No wonder that, faced with the choice between either white bread sandwiches or biscuits and cakes, people so often choose the biscuits or cakes.

Much of the wholemeal bread on the market nowadays is also pre-packed and sliced. It's made from wholegrain flour, of course, but it, too, is sophisticated with chemical additives – 'processing aids' and 'improvers' – that are good for business but not for you. One of the biggest favours you can do for yourself, in your progress from Fat

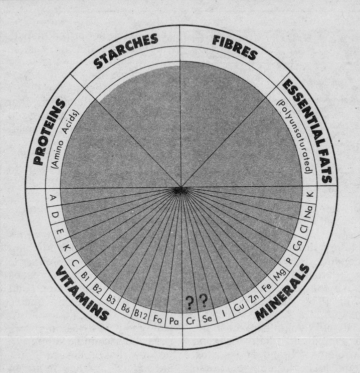

● **Fit sandwich bar lunch: fish and fresh vegetables.** If you can find a bar that serves selections of salads you are in luck. You can choose a near-perfect lunch to eat there or take away in little pots. This 700 calories of fresh vegetables in season, together with a couple of tasty sardines and a big roll, is super-rich in vitamins and minerals. (Menu: page 23. Recipe: page 158.)

to Fit, is to find shops that sell good old-fashioned wholemeal bread. It's easy to tell the difference. Plastic bread of all types, white, brown and wholemeal, can be squeezed almost to nothing in the packet.

Good wholemeal bread is made from wholegrain flour, water, salt and yeast, and that's all. Incidentally, the salt added to bread just by itself contains more than enough sodium for good health. Good wholemeal bread is solid;

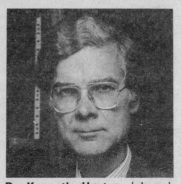

**Dr Kenneth Heaton** (above). Reader in Medicine at Bristol University, is an authority on dietary fibre and its health benefits. However, Dr Heaton is interested not just in fibre, but in food as a whole.

In 1983, he published the results of a study in which for six weeks volunteers ate either a wholefood diet, including wholemeal bread and pastas, with lots of vegetables and fruit, or else a 'refined' diet, including white bread, sugar and confectionery, in amounts typically eaten in Britain.

The key finding was that the people on the wholefood diet were a lot better nourished, with vitamins and minerals as well as fibre, yet at the same time were satisfied with fewer calories, and they lost weight.

Dr Heaton believes that highly concentrated, processed foods, and sugars in particular, trick people into consuming more calories than their bodies need. 'We are designed to chew our food,' he says. 'If we eat foods that don't need chewing, over-consumption is likely. The body is able to control its energy intake if we provide it with food in something approximating a natural state, but when processing increases the energy content of food and makes it easy to eat, the body's defences are not equipped to deal with it.' Dr Heaton's work gives solid scientific support to the view that processed foods, and sugars in particular, are an important cause of overweight and obesity, and he points out that 'this tendency is increased by the fact that sugar is often combined with fat in manufactured foods'.

you can't squeeze it. And it's very tasty. Shop around if you're lucky enough to have several small master bakers or wholefood shops and sandwich bars in your area. It's worth being as fussy and particular about bread as a careful shopper is about cuts of meat.

A high quality wholegrain sandwich, filled with tasty items, is one of the most delicious convenience foods ever devised. At the same time it's doing you good, by being so filling, and so full of whole starches, fibres, vitamins and minerals, together with proteins and essential fats.

Then there's that other ingenious invention, the little styrofoam pot. So instead of sandwiches, take away pots of home-made soup, hummous (chickpeas), or small, fresh salads to eat wherever you like. Salad doesn't have to mean rabbit food. Solid salads are just the stuff for people who want to lose excess fat. Look at the Wheel of the second Fit lunch, shown on page 27. Delicious and filling in summer or winter, it's a mixture of filling ingredients (potatoes and butter beans, both with a little dressing) and of whatever takes your fancy – the choice here is celery, mushrooms, tomato and a parsley garnish.

A couple of sardines make this takeaway even more tasty. There's no need to spread fat on the wholemeal roll: the fish and the salad dressing provide quite enough juice. Afterwards, to eat straight away or as a little treat in the afternoon, there are two whole fruits. Select whatever you most like, in season. It's worth knowing, though, that some popular fruits, apples in particular, have had a lot of goodness and taste bred out of them, as fruit farmers search for the 'perfect' (meaning big, uniform and watery) product.

What this Wheel doesn't show is that this salad lunch, perfect for picnics as well as days at the office, is 'super-rich' in many vitamins and minerals. For example, it contains in its 700 calories more than a day's worth of vitamin C and calcium, and is also very rich in essential fats. You will have noticed that both of the Fit sandwich bar lunches shown here include fish. The fact is that fish that swim in the deep sea, such as tuna and sardines, as well as herring, mackerel and other oily fish, are bulging with goodness. If you don't like fish, lean meats or poultry are alternatives. If you don't eat meat or fish? No problem. If you took away the sardines and instead added more potatoes and beans, or lentils, and bread, together with the other salad items, you'd still have a pretty full Wheel●

# TWENTY-FIVE YEARS ON A YO-YO

Looking back and thinking about it now, I realize that I worried about my weight (meaning my fat), for twenty-five years. In 1950, fizz and chips was the 'in thing' for kids at the Ambler Road primary school (London N4), as we dawdled home after school. I became a plump little chap.

Age twelve, at secondary school in the country, I went on my first calorie-cutting diet, and in the twelve weeks of an autumn term was down from eight to seven stone. The school doctor, who ceremonially weighed all the young boys in the school at the beginning and end of term, was furious. My weight was the only line on his graph that went down, not up. In those days thriving meant rising lines on height and weight graphs.

Age thirty-seven I had a weighing machine of my very own. For a quarter of a century my weight had yo-yo'd up, and then down (on a calorie-cutting diet), and up and down (a new diet), and up. Spending your life on or between low-calorie diet regimes is no fun. Few clothes fit. You fear food. For me, what I hated most was the sense of being out of control. Getting fat was a dirty little secret that I couldn't keep to myself, because it showed. I lost self-respect: no matter how I might shine in other areas of my life, I felt inferior, degraded.

So I followed the diet in vogue – high protein, low carbohydrate, low fat, Stillman, Scarsdale, Atkins, Yudkin. They all amounted to the same instruction: cut calories to 1,000 – 1,500 a day and you'll eventually get in trim.

Then, one year in the late 1970s, everything changed for me. One day I realized that I was eating and drinking whatever I enjoyed and was staying at a steady weight. The difference was that I had started to run, slowly but regularly, and that after a long holiday in Greece, I had taken to a Mediterranean diet. But I wasn't eating any less food. Quite the reverse; as far as I could tell, I was eating more. In 1981, during a month in California, I found out why the dieting books had got it wrong.

I was on a visit to San Francisco and, in between jogging over the Golden Gate bridge, I was visiting Stanford University: in particular, Professor Peter Wood, deputy director of the Heart Disease Prevention Program Unit. Dr Wood is English by birth and, like his colleagues, Professors Jack Farquhar, Bill Haskell and Ralph Paffenbarger, a champion of exercise and of good eating. What the team at Stanford had found out was that regular, vigorous exercise of the type now known as 'aerobic' is of far greater value than the old textbooks say.

The result of such exercise is that your body speeds up at all times so that it burns up more fuel from food not only when you are exercising, but also when you are sleeping – and eating! Dr Wood pointed out that middle-aged women who played energetic tennis regularly were lean, yet were consuming around 1,000 calories more than their overweight, sedentary neighbours.

I then found out, from a search of the scientific literature, that studies carried out since the beginning of the twentieth century show that when people go on calorie-cutting diets, their bodies slow down. *You* can tell the difference between going on a diet, and famine or starvation, but your body cannot; it adapts to protect you by making do with less food and also preserving that part of you most needed in times of famine – fat. People who continually go on calorie-cutting diets are turning themselves into human versions of the camel.

With Hetty Einzig, I wrote about these findings in an earlier book, *Dieting Makes You Fat.* My own twenty-five years on a yo-yo were over, and in the last few years I've been delighted to hear from readers who have at last found the way to be free from semi-starvation diet regimes, and who are enjoying their food for the first time in their adult lives●

# READY AND STEADY TO GO

Now you are ready to start your journey from Fat to Fit. This is the first of eight chapters showing you how to make the plan work, from breakfast, to snacks, to simple lunches and suppers, to dinner parties. After that, starting on page 155, you can put the entire plan together, for a whole day's and week's meals, at all seasons of the year.

And a big plus: every part of the plan is complete in itself. Dip into it and get to work. But first, before you start, here are a set of questions for you to answer. If you have access to a copying machine, you might like to take extra copies of this page and keep a record over the months.

It's easy to take your pulse rate at rest: a good time is while lying in bed or sitting in a chair in the morning. Your doctor will take your blood pressure on request and should tell you the result: ask for both the systolic and diastolic pressures, written as (for example) 120/80, or 125/90.

| Age | Height | Weight |
|---|---|---|
| Chest | Waist | Hips |
| Pulse rate at rest | | Blood pressure |

Rate the following things about yourself (tick a box)

| | Great | Good | OK | Bad | Awful |
|---|---|---|---|---|---|
| Health | | | | | |
| Fitness | | | | | |
| Self-respect | | | | | |
| General mood | | | | | |
| Energy | | | | | |

# FAT TO FIT

## 2

# A HEARTY BREAKFAST

**W**hat's the first thing you do in the morning if you want to lose fat? Skip breakfast, right? . . . Wrong! The first step from FAT TO FIT is to enjoy a nourishing and filling breakfast ● Professor Philip James of the NACNE report explains what's special about starchy food ● Why recovering 300 calories of lost activity can make all the difference between Fat and Fit ● And a special quiz for you to fill out and keep to check your progress, on food and mood. What's a treat for you? Sweets, sausages, or fruit?

So you really do want to get rid of that extra flab. You're reading this book to pick up some tips, but you're sceptical because you've looked through calorie-cutting diet plans in the past and maybe tried some out – but the extra flab is still there. Never mind (you may be thinking) – every diet plan has a gimmick and maybe the gimmick of FAT TO FIT will suit me. Give it a whirl.

People who try to lose extra fat are always trained to believe in certain ideas which all amount to fear of food. They think of food as some kind of enemy. People who read diet books are given the idea that if they're disobedient and don't do exactly what the diet doctor or expert tells them, they'll swell into balloons. Much like Victorian fathers, diet doctors are very keen to tell you that it is Good to feel hungry. After all, if you are fat, you are Bad. You deserve to suffer because you have been greedy, and that's a sin. So dieters are encouraged to hate their bodies and to submit themselves to rituals of self-denial, just like religious fanatics.

Sounds familiar? 'It's always best', diet doctors say primly, 'to get up from a meal feeling a little hungry.' But beliefs such as these are, literally, un-natural. Throughout history, people have eaten their fill and enjoyed food and, throughout history, few people have become fat. In every society, great days are feast days. For thousands of years, growing, harvesting, preparing and eating food has been a central part of human culture. It's only in this century that many people have become over-fat.

Fat people do not eat more than thin people, as a rule. Rather, most people in Britain eat the wrong kind of food. The typical British food supply, heavy in saturated fats and added sugars, makes some people ill and other people fat. What is also true is that most of us, dieters especially, have got the wrong idea about food. Part of the purpose of FAT TO FIT is to encourage you to enjoy your food and to eat your fill – maybe for the first time in your adult life.

Take breakfast. The trouble for most over-fat people starts at the beginning of the day: they don't take breakfast. They leave it. When I was on a diet I never ate breakfast, because I'm not hungry first thing in the morning. It never occurred to me that my craving for confectionery (always resisted, often without success), that started around eleven o'clock in the morning, was because I hadn't eaten any breakfast.

Do yourself a favour. In this chapter I'll show how to enjoy a good, simple, warming, filling and nourishing breakfast.

The quality of three breakfasts, all supplying 400 calories, is revealed by the three Wheels of Health on pages

# THE CHOICE IS YOURS

**BREAKFAST**
(photographs: pages 100, 101)

| | FAT<br>400 calories | FIT (1)<br>400 calories | FIT (2)<br>400 calories |
|---|---|---|---|
| | Cornflakes (1 oz), sugar (1 tsp), full fat milk | Muesli base (2 oz), dates (1 oz), fresh fruit, skimmed milk | Plain yoghurt (6 oz, pear, raisins (½ oz) |
| | Toast (white, 1 slice), butter, marmalade | | Wholemeal toast (2 slices), tomatoes (2), corn oil (½ tsp) |
| | Coffee (1 cup), sugar (1 tsp), full fat milk | Tea (1 cup), skimmed milk | Tea (1 cup), skimmed milk |
| | | fresh fruit | Apricots (3½ oz) |
| Saturated fats | HEAVY | LIGHT | LIGHT |
| Sugars | HEAVY | LIGHT | LIGHT |
| Salt | HEAVY | LIGHT | LIGHT |
| Additives | MEDIUM | LIGHT | LIGHT |
| Proteins | RICH | RICH | RICH |
| Starches | POOR/MEDIUM | MEDIUM | POOR |
| Fibres | POOR | RICH | SUPER-RICH |
| Essential fats | POOR | POOR/MEDIUM | RICH |
| Vitamin A | POOR | POOR | RICH |
| Vitamin $B_1$ | SUPER-RICH | RICH | RICH |
| Potassium (K) | POOR | RICH | RICH |
| Magnesium (Mg) | POOR | RICH | RICH |

Key to terms used here and on Wheels of Health: page 199.
Breakfast recipes: Chapter 9.

36, 37 and 39 – two of these breakfasts are pictured on pages 100–101. The first thing to be said about the Fat breakfast on page 100, typical of what millions of people in Britain have got used to in the last twenty years or so, is that it's not all bad. Ready-to-eat breakfast cereals, like corn flakes, include a few vitamins added back by the manufacturers as well as some proteins, starches and fibres, and full-fat milk is a good source of calcium (Ca).

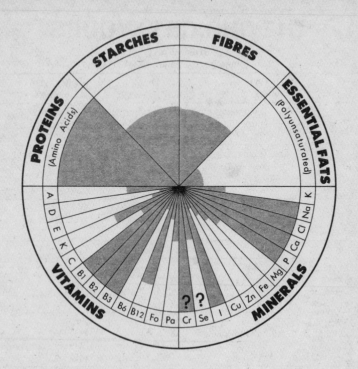

● **Fat breakfast; processed cereal plus fats and sugars.** Ready-to-eat breakfast cereals and white toast are not all bad. They have some starches and fibres as well as protein and are 'fortified' with vitamins B1, B2, B3, and the minerals calcium (Ca) and iron (Fe). But there's a heavy price to pay: chemical additives, mostly in the bread, salt, and saturated fats and sugars. (Photograph: page 100. Menu: page 35.)

White sliced bread, ready for toasting, contains lots of calcium (in the form of added chalk), and some of vitamins $B_1$ and $B_3$, also iron (Fe), lost during manufacture but added back afterwards.

But there is a heavy price to pay for what goodness there is in this breakfast, in the form of chemical additives, saturated fats (in the milk, and butter) and sugars (in the marmalade, and added to the corn flakes and coffee). The

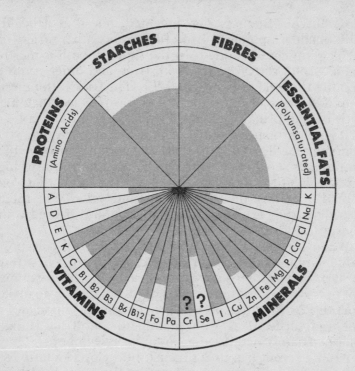

● **Fit breakfast: muesli with fruit.** Most supermarkets stock sugar-free muesli. Better still, buy your own muesli base and add lots of sliced whole fruits, a little dried fruit. On a winter's morning try a big bowl of porridge – a hot version of muesli. Like the Fat breakfast opposite this is 400 calories, but is filling and nourishing. (Photograph: page 101. Menu: page 35. Recipe: page 158.)

result is a meal short of many vitamins and minerals.

The first Fit breakfast, shown here, is just as ready to eat as any packaged breakfast cereal. It's muesli, invented in the 1930s by a Swiss and for many years only available at high prices in health food stores. You can now buy muesli at any supermarket, but be sure to buy the sugar-free type made from whole grains. The packaged products are heavy in added sugars and are also more expensive.

Dr Bircher-Benner, who invented muesli as a health cure, made it up mainly from fresh fruit with a variety of wholegrain cereals added. In the shops, muesli is mostly made from cereal with dried fruit and nuts, simply because these have a long shelf-life. The trick with muesli is to add lots of fresh fruit of your own choice, together with a small sprinkling of dried fruit and/or nuts, to taste.

It's worth taking trouble to find the mixture that you and your family find most tempting, and if you serve the ingredients separately, your family can have fun working out the mixture they like best. As a slimmer, what you should watch is the dried fruit and nuts. Use them sparingly: they are very nourishing but also packed with energy (calories).

When you think about it, muesli is a type of cold porridge. Grandmother may have told you that the best way to start a cold winter's day was with a big bowl of steaming hot porridge. Grandmother was right, but the way to make porridge extra nutritious is to avoid adding white sugar or salt and, instead, as with muesli, to add fruit (I like chopped dates), or a few nuts, or just a little honey.

After a recent trip to Sri Lanka, I developed a taste for jaggery, a hard raw dark brown distillation of sweetness made from certain types of palm tree, marvellously intense in flavour and delicious flaked from the block. Like jaggery, raw brown sugar should be fragrant, rich in minerals, and is fine used sparingly just as a relish. But make sure it's the real thing: look for an ingredients label guaranteeing a high mineral content.

If you like milk with porridge, use skimmed milk, which has the goodness of full-fat milk without the saturated fats and is cheaper. Alternatively, try lemon juice with honey, which is my favourite. Scots disapprove of all these diversions and real porridge enthusiasts eat it just as it comes.

A lot of the proteins, starches and fibres in the second Fit breakfast, shown here, come from the wholemeal toast. If the slices are thick, the 'starches' segment of the Wheel

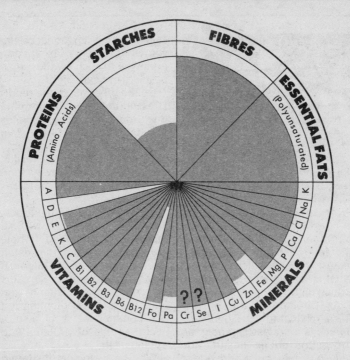

● **Fit breakfast: savoury toast with fruit.** Everything depends on the quality of the bread and what you put on it. Wholemeal bread is rich in B vitamins and plenty of minerals. Tomatoes, grilled, or fried in a little high quality oil, add vitamins A, C and E and essential fats. And a plain low-fat yoghurt, with fruits, for calcium (Ca) and potassium (K). Yet this is still only 400 calories! (Menu: page 35. Recipe: page 160.)

will be full (in which case, leave out the dried fruit from the yoghurt). The secret with toast is to find delicious and nutritious toppings. Tomatoes, grilled, or fried in a little high-quality oil, are a favourite of mine. Olive oil is a good alternative to high-polyunsaturated oils. You will have been told that fried food is Out. On the whole this is good advice. Breakfast fry-ups, swimming in lard, are of course very fattening and also a way to an early grave. There's

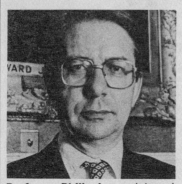

**Professor Philip James** (above) is now the best-known nutritionist in Britain. He was the man behind NACNE, the expert report which showed what is wrong with the typical British diet.

As Director of the Rowett Research Institute in Aberdeen, James is a tireless campaigner for better public health, not only in Britain, but worldwide.

He was Secretary of the Royal College of Physicians' working party on obesity, whose 1983 report made the sharpest possible distinction between starches and sugars. Of processed sugar, the report said 'sugar is an unnecessary source of energy in a community with such a widespread problem of overweight'.

On the other hand, the report stressed that the old slimming book idea, that carbohydrates are fattening, is just plain wrong. Everybody, including people who are over-fat, should eat more starchy food like bread, cereals, potatoes and pastas.

Above all other staple foods, 'Obesity' and the NACNE report recommended whole grain cereal, most readily eaten in the form of wholemeal bread. In whole form, cereal is rich not only in starch and fibre, but also in B vitamins and many minerals; it is also a useful source of proteins and essential fats.

Why have doctors in Britain been so slow to share the good news about starchy foods? Dr James does not mince his words. 'The nutritionally most ignorant professional group is probably the medical profession.'

nothing wrong, however, with using the frying pan for little delicacies like tomatoes. Just don't fry in grease.

Another favourite of mine, on toast, is olive paste, which is deep green in colour and has a wonderful aroma on the hot bread. You may be able to find it in your supermarket; it's rather salty, although not as salty as branded yeast or meat/vegetable spreads.

Consider the difference between white bread or toast

spread with butter or margarine, with jam or marmalade on top, and wholemeal bread or toast, cut thick with a nourishing treat on top. You don't have to speculate about the difference: it's shown by the contrast between the two Wheels of Health on pages 36 and 39.

Savoury toppings are generally the best choice for breakfast toast. One sweet Fit choice is roasted sesame seeds with just enough honey on the toast to stop the seeds sliding off.

In Chapter 6 I'll be showing you the difference between Fat and Fit cooked breakfasts, to enjoy at weekends, or as 'brunch' in the middle of the day with friends. Meanwhile, what other treats can you enjoy, as a slimmer, for a quick and simple breakfast?

Yoghurt is always a good choice. Like skimmed milk, low-fat yoghurt has the nourishment of full-fat milk – calcium (Ca) in particular – without the saturated fats. Live yoghurt is always best: grow your own or buy it in good supermarkets. Some yoghurts are fatty: Greek yoghurts made from sheeps' milk, for example, contain between five and ten per cent fat. Any full-fat yoghurt, whether made from cows', sheep's or goats' milk, should be eaten only as a treat. Forget about the sweetened and chemicalized 'fruit' yoghurts. The best Fit choice for everyday is low-fat yoghurt, eaten either by itself or else made really tasty with sliced-up fresh fruits.

Fat breakfast tables are laid with a sugar-bowl and a salt-pot. Kick these off your table and out of your life. A Fit breakfast table is laid with a bowl of whole fruits in season. If you've got the time to sit and chat over breakfast, peel yourself an orange, or cut up an apple or pear, or have some grapes – whatever you enjoy most. If you live near a street market, you are in luck. I live just up the road from West London's Portobello Road market. In season the stalls are glorious with the colour and variety of fruits. If you get the chance try fresh mango, guava, lychee, kiwi fruit, passion fruit, or figs. Be adventurous.

# STOKE UP ON STARCH

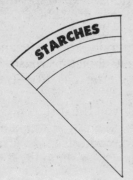

STARCHES

Everybody must have heard by now that it's a good idea, for health, to eat lots of starchy food. The prospect sounds unattractive. 'Sugar' is a term of affection; no boy ever called his girl 'starch'. As food, starch sounds much the same as stodge: without colour or flavour and, surely, fattening? So what's so special about starch?

Since the beginning of recorded history, and before, the staple food on which almost all settled communities in the world have depended has been some form of cereal. All people who have moved from nomadic life to some form of agriculture have grown and developed a staple grain with which to make bread or an equivalent food. In the East this grain is rice; in South America, corn; in some parts of Africa, sorghum or millet. In Britain and other Western countries staple grains have been rye, oats and barley as well as wheat. In modern times wheat has become the dominant cereal.

Since the development of agriculture, up to 10,000 years ago, most people, most of the time, have relied on cereal foods, together with root and other vegetables and certain fruits, to supply around three quarters of their energy needs. Before agriculture there is good evidence that people were rather more gatherers than hunters, not so much meat as root and fruit eaters.

What most cereals have in common with some vegetables

Peaches and apricots are both superb sources of vitamin A and English favourites are good in season: gooseberries, plums, damsons, strawberries, raspberries, blackberries.

Eat as much fresh fruit as you like for breakfast. Get into the habit of taking fruit to work, or putting some by for later in the morning. Be adventurous. You never know what a new and exotic fruit tastes like until you've tried it.

With breakfast, as with all meals, the foods to avoid are

like potatoes and beans is that most of their energy is supplied by starch, also known chemically as 'polysaccharides' or, in America, as 'complex carbohydrates'.

The value of cereals and other starchy foods in whole form is that the starch comes in a very nourishing package. Whole wheat grain, for example, is a good source of fibre, vitamins and minerals (from the bran and outer layers), and of protein (from the white inner endosperm). It isn't a complete food – no one food is – but made into bread, whole grain deserves the name 'the staff of life'.

Whole fresh potatoes are also full of nourishment (including vitamin C, not found in grain), and beans, lentils and similar foods, fresh or dried, are a rich yet cheap source of protein.

What's gone wrong with food in Western countries within the last half a dozen generations since industrialization is that much starchy food has been replaced, as a source of energy, by processed fatty and sugary food. Only about one quarter of calories in the British food supply today come as starch.

Filling up on starchy foods in whole form, above all at breakfast time, is not only good for health, but also good advice for everybody who wants to lose fat. Many slimmers fear food and most slimmers fear feeling full, but a satisfying and nourishing meal first thing is the best guard against cravings later on.

Because a healthy – and Fit – diet cuts right down on the foods that supply calories with little or no nourishment, it's a diet that's rich in whole, starchy food. To fill the starch segment in the Wheel of Health, shown above, the target is to double the average consumption of wholemeal bread, cereals and pastas, potatoes and all other nourishing starchy foods, so that they supply at least a half of all your calories.

highly processed products and any other foods heavy in saturated fats, and/or added sugars, and/or salt, and/or additives. It's also a good time to eat lots of wholegrain cereals, in the form of bread, porridge or muesli.

Above all, enjoy a hearty breakfast. The habit of skipping breakfast can be quite hard to break, but it's worth it. After a while, you'll stop having cravings for sweet things half-way through the morning. You'll be less

43

# INTOLERANCE

Some food makes some people ill. It's now well-known that the two most common problem foods are cows' milk and wheat. Many people react to these foods as if they are poisons. Terms used for these conditions include lactose intolerance (milk), and gluten intolerance or coeliac disease (wheat).

So what do you do if you have a problem with milk and/or wheat? What options, for example, do you have for breakfast?

First, some people react as if poisoned, not to the milk or wheat itself, but to contaminants – traces of chemicals, like pesticides sprayed on wheat, or bleaches used in white bread. They are, indeed, being poisoned. Try going organic: find milk from a wholefood shop and eat genuine wholemeal bread.

Second, the reason why many people are, in effect, poisoned by milk and/or wheat probably dates back to when they were little babies. The immune system of infants is immature. If weaning on to cows' milk and solids happens too early, the baby's body is liable to react against milk and cereal proteins, rejecting them as 'foreign'. Once learned, this reaction can persist throughout life.

The lesson for mothers is that breast is best and don't be hurried into introducing baby to solids. If, as an adult, you can't take cows' milk or wheat, try goats' or sheep's milk and other cereals, such as rye and the oats that make porridge. This often works: rejection can be highly selective, fortunately.

Whole starchy food is such a valuable and economical staple that it's worth persisting, and finding a cereal that suits you. And it's not difficult to construct a healthy diet without milk.

For further advice, contact: Action Against Allergy, 43, The Downs, Wimbledon, London SW20 8HG, enclosing a large s.a.e.

inclined to think 'Oh, to hell with it' and over-eat at supper time; you'll start the day feeling good, just like you did when you were a child. With good food inside, you may even look forward to a walk at lunchtime or to the shops. Here are the things to remember for the beginning of the day:

● Start your day right with a good breakfast.
● Enjoy being satisfied by nourishing food.
● Never be tempted to go to work feeling hungry.
● Look forward to good food and fresh air.

# IT ALL ADDS UP

Since the turn of the century we in Britain, as a nation, have eaten less and less food and yet become fatter and fatter. The reason, quite simply, is that as a nation we have become physically inactive. The same is true of people in all Western and Westernized countries.

So why doesn't everybody get fat? Simple. We are all born different. Everybody has different strong points and weak points. Not everybody suffers from a sedentary life. Of three inactive women, one may get fat, another may develop weak and brittle bones as she gets older, and the third may apparently be unaffected. To use an apt, old-fashioned word, we have different constitutions.

All the same though, almost every sedentary person puts on excess and unsightly flab in adult life. And plenty of underweight people are over-fat. It's probable that most people in Britain would like to lose some fat.

So what's the best way to get rid of it? Recent studies have begun to recommend vigorous exercise, especially dance-exercise, 'aerobics', jogging and long-distance running. You may have read features in women's and fitness magazines along these lines – I've written some myself! And yes, it is true that anybody who takes plenty of exercise will lose fat and gain fitness and health.

But don't run before you walk. Before you start investing in leotards, trainers or club subscriptions, take a good look at the amount of activity, as distinct from exercise, you already do in your everyday life. For example, our grandparents didn't go for 'the burn' nor did they run marathons. Throughout history people have preferred to take it easy when they can. Our problem is that machines have taken over our lives to an un-natural extent.

In the last century, or even in the early years of this one, our grandparents walked a lot more than we do. Children walked to and from school; housewives to the shops, and

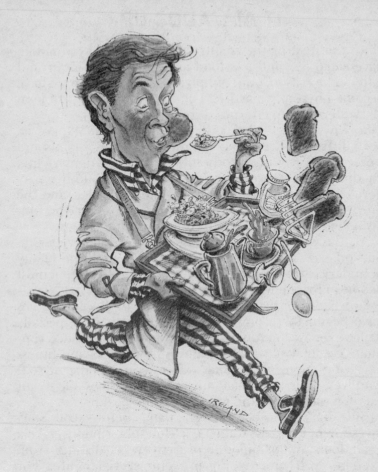

back again laden with shopping; men and women to and from work. At home, women cooked and cleaned and men worked in the garden or allotment, using simple tools.

Now, much work is done for us; all we do is flick a switch or press a button. Cars have replaced walking. Vegetables are chopped with magic mixers, lawns cut with motor mowers. Household appliances are advertised as 'labour-saving', food, as 'convenient'. In conquering drudgery, we are in danger of falling into a state of physical disuse and premature decay.

Contemporary estimates show that before the age of the car, people probably used something like one seventh, or about fifteen per cent, more energy than people today. A woman nowadays who is in 'energy balance', neither gaining nor losing weight, will be consuming, and also using, somewhere around 2,000 calories a day. The corresponding figure for women of fifty years ago was around 2,300.

For men, of course, the figures are higher and amount to somewhere around 2,600 calories a day now, compared with 3,000 calories a day fifty years ago. What these round-figure averages show is that our grandparents ate and used something like 300–400 calories a day more than we do. To put it another way, a woman of fifty years ago who consumed 2,300 calories a day was generally unlikely to become fat, whereas a woman who consumes 2,300 calories a day now, is fairly likely to put on weight.

The FAT TO FIT plan is designed to show you how you can put those missing 300–400 calories a day back into your everyday life. How you do this is up to you. If your choice is vigorous exercise, and you decide to get into training, then half an hour a day of vigorous dancing, running or swimming will do the trick. But what you can also do is to build activity into your life by making the kind of changes that any able-bodied person can make

For example, scientists reckon that manual typing uses 0.2 calories a minute more than electric typing – the difference between banging and touching the keys. This piffling difference adds up to fifty calories in the day of a secretary who types for four hours. Suppose the same secretary also walks half an hour a day, to and from a healthy sandwich bar lunch, rather than sitting in a canteen: that's an extra 100 calories. If she also walks up stairs for a total of five minutes a day, rather than taking a lift, that's an extra twenty-five calories. These three simple choices add up to 175 calories a day, which takes you more than half way to the target of 300 extra calories a day. It all adds up

# YOUR FOOD AND YOUR MOOD

Likes and dislikes about food can go back to childhood. Parents often reward their children with confectionery. If you were given chocolate and sweets as a reward when you were young, it's quite likely that as an adult you'll think to yourself 'well, I've been really good; let's just have a little sweet thing', maybe as you're buying a newspaper or waiting in the supermarket line. The childhood memory lives on.

There again, likes and dislikes can be based on misinformation. For decades, slimmers have been told that starchy foods are fattening. People who are trying to lose fat still say 'no thanks' to bread and potatoes, but will eat fatty cheese.

As you start to go from Fat to Fit, record your feelings for the following foods. Please don't tick the box you think you *ought* to tick. Just think of the food, see how you feel about it and record that feeling. If you have access to a copying machine, you might like to take extra copies of this page and keep a record over the months. We'll be repeating this quiz later in the plan.

|  | Love | Like | OK | Dislike | Hate |
|---|---|---|---|---|---|
| Beans | | | | | |
| Biscuits | | | | | |
| Bread | | | | | |
| Confectionery | | | | | |
| Crisps | | | | | |
| Fish | | | | | |
| Fruit | | | | | |
| Meat | | | | | |
| Salad | | | | | |
| Sausages | | | | | |
| Soft Drinks | | | | | |
| Vegetables | | | | | |

# FAT to FIT

## 3

# EATING TOGETHER

**C**alorie-cutting dieters have a miserable, lonely life: they lose out on all the pleasures of sharing meals at home ● There's no calorie-cutting as you go from Fat to Fit. Better news still, a supper that makes you Fit can be twice the size of a supper that makes you Fat ● Dr Denis Burkitt tells the story of the high-fibre revolution ● Why our average daily activity is peanuts – and how to recover that lost energy. Once you've got some activity back into your life, you can keep going longer – and yes, that does mean making love!

Faced with a meal at home, what do dieters say? Have you ever been on a calorie-cutting diet? Do you remember saying things like 'No thanks, really, I'm not hungry'. Or 'I had such a big meal at lunchtime, I'm quite full'. Or 'You eat it, I couldn't manage any more'. Or 'Mmm, that was good' (pushing away a still full plate) 'but it was so filling'. Sounds familiar?

Lies! People on semi-starvation diets are hungry most of the time (surprise, surprise!). In public, they pretend to have a tiny appetite; at home, they avoid the pleasure and the company of shared meals and act as if ill. In private, though, the cravings of hunger overpower the intention to starve, so it's round the corner to the newsagents ('just out for a moment, won't be long') or upstairs to the back of the bedroom wardrobe ('just going to look for something'), for a quick fix of confectionery. It's clever stuff, confectionery. It's very more-ish, as you may have noticed, or as scientists would say, addictive.

It's a miserable, furtive business, going on a diet, and evenings can be the worst time of all. Evenings are the time when the people who share a home are together. The evening meal, however simple, can be an occasion to share news, make plans, and enjoy the company of your family. Dieters cut themselves off from all that. Avoiding meals, especially the evening meal, is like banishing yourself from society.

So now, here is the good news for everybody who wants to lose that excess fat, but also wants to keep friends, family, health and sanity. Meals are all part of the FAT TO FIT plan. More than that, in following the plan you should gradually become slimmer, while at the same time eating bigger meals. Filling yourself up, and enjoying an evening meal, is all part of the deal.

Let me explain. 'Big' and 'small', used of food, have different meanings which are muddled up in dieting books. A big meal can mean a meal heavy in calories (energy), or it can mean a meal heavy in weight. In practice, these are very different meanings. Likewise, a small meal can mean a meal that supplies little energy (calories), or a meal that takes up little space on the plate. These, too, are very different things.

Take the two evening meals whose menus are opposite, pictured on pages 102–103. On the left, there's chop, chips and peas, followed by apple crumble and custard. On the right, there's chicken risotto, followed by stewed fruit and yoghurt. Both meals include meat, vegetables and fruit. Both supply the same amount of energy: 900 calories.

The chicken meal is much bigger. It takes up more

# THE CHOICE IS YOURS

## SUPPER AT HOME

| | FAT<br>900 calories | FIT (1)<br>900 calories | FIT (2)<br>900 calories |
|---|---|---|---|
| | Chop (5oz, grilled)<br>Chips (3oz, fried in corn oil)<br>Peas (2oz, boiled) | Chicken (3½oz, boiled)<br>Brown rice (3½oz, boiled)<br>Onion (2oz), green pepper (2oz), tomato (3½oz), almonds (½oz) (all fried in corn oil)<br>Sweet corn (2oz) boiled<br>Green salad (3½oz) | Liver (5½oz, fried)<br>Noodles (2oz)<br>French beans (4oz), onions (4oz), cauliflower (3oz), carrots (3oz), broccoli (3½oz) (all stir-fried in corn oil) |
| | Apple crumble (packet, 2oz)<br>Custard (packet, 1oz) | Stewed fruit (6oz in total, apples, pears, apricot)<br>Yoghurt (3oz, plain) | Strawberries (3½oz), banana (½), in yoghurt (plain, 3oz) and white wine (½ glass) |
| Saturated fats<br>Sugars<br>Salt<br>Additives | HEAVY<br>HEAVY<br>HEAVY*<br>MEDIUM | LIGHT<br>LIGHT<br>LIGHT**<br>LIGHT | LIGHT<br>LIGHT<br>LIGHT**<br>LIGHT |
| Proteins<br>Starches<br>Fibres<br>Essential fats | RICH<br>POOR<br>POOR/MEDIUM<br>RICH | SUPER-RICH<br>MEDIUM<br>RICH<br>SUPER-RICH | SUPER-RICH<br>POOR<br>RICH<br>SUPER-RICH |
| Vitamin A<br>Vitamin $B_{12}$ | POOR<br>SUPER-RICH | RICH<br>MEDIUM | SUPER-RICH<br>SUPER-RICH |
| Magnesium (Mg)<br>Iron (Fe) | POOR<br>POOR | RICH<br>MEDIUM | RICH<br>SUPER-RICH |

* if added    ** if not added

Key to terms used here and on Wheels of Health: page 199.
Fit supper recipes: Chapter 9.

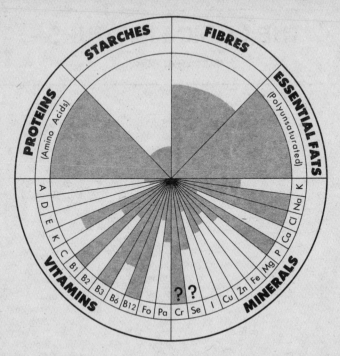

● **Fat supper: Chop, chips and peas, and crumble.** There's no such thing as a meal that is all bad. Meat (in this case pork or lamb) is rich in proteins, B vitamins and some minerals. Peas are a good source of fibre and corn oil is polyunsaturated. But the meal is patchy in its supply of vitamins and minerals because of the saturated fats and sugars in it. And it may leave you hungry. (Photograph: page 102. Menu: page 51.)

room on the plate. It weighs twice as much as the chop meal. Every gram of the chop meal contains over two calories. By contrast, there is only one calorie in every gram of the chicken meal.

The chop meal is concentrated in calories because of the fats in the chop and chips, and the fats and sugars in the apple crumble. The chicken meal is much more bulky because of the water and fibres in the rice, vegetables and

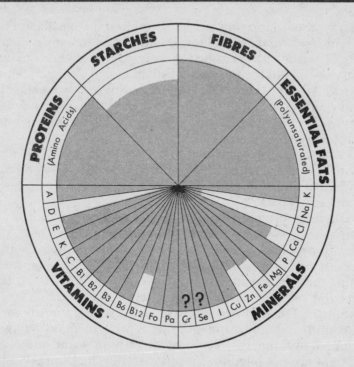

● **Fit supper: Chicken risotto, and stewed fruit.** This makes a much more nourishing meal. It's made with four ounces of chicken and four ounces of rice per person. The vegetables and fruit are rich in vitamins A, C and E. Brown rice, like all whole grains, is rich in B vitamins, minerals and trace elements. This supper is also twice the size of the Fat supper. (Photograph: page 103. Menu: page 51. Recipe: page 159.)

fruit. Also, the balance between meat and vegetables is different in the two meals. The five ounces of chop (per person) is accompanied by the same weight of chips and peas. By contrast, four ounces of chicken in the risotto gives savour to four times its weight in rice and vegetables. (The four ounces of dry rice per person will take up its own weight in water when boiled.)

If you like meat and poultry, part of the secret is to

change the balance in your food between the meat and the cereal foods and vegetables. Do what the Italians do: eat lots of pasta with meat just to taste. Do what the Indians do: ask for double portions of plain boiled rice with your curry. All over the world, country people enjoy meat, fish and poultry, but flesh dominates their meals only on feast days. Throughout history, everyday food has been mainly staple cereals with vegetables.

Of course, the meal that takes up more space on the plate also takes up more space in your stomach. It's filling and satisfying. The chicken risotto meal is unlikely to leave you feeling 'peckish'.

It is also very much more nourishing than the chop and chips meal, as you can see by looking at the two Wheels of Health on pages 52–53. Everything in the chicken risotto meal is of high quality. The problem with the chop and chips meal is that its goodness is rather overwhelmed by fats and sugars and this immediately shows in the Wheel. Saturated fats and processed sugars are heavy in calories but empty of nourishment; this is why so many of the segments of the Fat meal showing vitamin and mineral content are not filled in. By contrast, the chicken risotto is almost a perfect meal.

Another good form of meat for a Fit meal is offal. When I was a small boy in the late 1940s, living in London's East End, offal meats were a great favourite for supper. My grandmother, like all the housewives in the neighbourhood, was an expert in the selection and cooking of meals of liver, kidneys, heart, brains and other rather more mysterious items, like 'lights', and sweetbreads. I never got to like tripe, cow-heel or pigs' trotters, but many of the vital organs of animals are really delicious.

What's more, liver and kidneys in particular are super-nutritious. Nowadays they are harder to find in the shops. A lot of the best bits of meat are thought of as rather unmentionable and are ground into food for dogs and

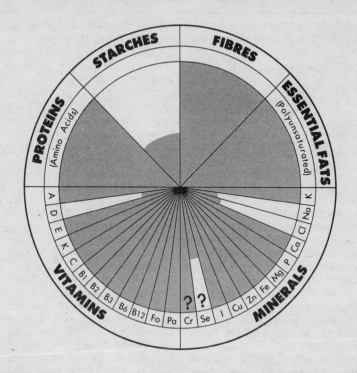

**● Fit supper: Liver and veg stir-fry, potatoes, greens, and summer salad.** This monster supper contains 900 calories, just like the other suppers. The liver and vegetables together are a spectacular source of many vitamins and minerals. Afterwards you can treat yourself to fruit in season, with a little yoghurt and white wine to taste, all blended in a delicious fruit fool. (Menu: page 51. Recipe: page 163.)

cats, which may be why our pets have shiny coats while we get dandruff.

There are all sorts of ways of cooking offal. A particularly delicious method is stir-frying, Chinese style. The secret is to cut up the meat and lots of vegetables quite small, and fry them in a thick pan in a very little hot oil. A frying-pan will do; a Chinese wok is better.

The result is a piping hot, crispy supper, super-rich in

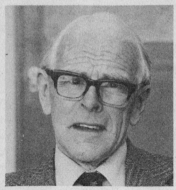

**Dr Denis Burkitt** (above) is the man who has put fibre on the world map, as a key part of any good diet. For the last fifteen years he has lectured widely and written one popular book (*Don't Forget Fibre in Your Diet*), always with the same message. Everybody will do well to eat lots of whole, fibre-rich food.

'Until the 1970s, experts thought fibre wasn't important. It was called "roughage". Nobody knew much about what it did and so nutritionists threw it out. The millers looked on bran almost as a contaminant. I still keep a press release, put out by the milling industry in 1972, stating that anybody who thought that fibre was important in food was "totally mistaken".'

Working as a surgeon in East Africa for years, Dr Burkitt began to suspect that many Western diseases and disorders were in part caused by the food we eat. Africans who eat traditional food are mostly free of such diseases.

The key factor, says Denis Burkitt, is fibre. Lack of fibre 'is the major reason why we in Britain, in common with other Western countries, are a constipated nation'. He is also sure that whole fibre-rich food can help you lose weight.

Dr Burkitt once proved his point with his famous 'Galway experiment'. Twenty-three young men from that county in his native Ireland ate two pounds of potatoes every day for three months. As soon as they had eaten the potatoes they were allowed to eat anything else they fancied. After three months, most had lost weight.

almost all the vitamins and minerals, and remarkably low in calories. A good accompaniment is a couple of potatoes, boiled in their skins, or baked, together with whatever green vegetables you like, steamed or boiled lightly in its own juices.

One of the big differences between the Fat chop'n'chips supper, and the two Fit suppers shown here, is that the proportions of meat to vegetables is different, as you can see by looking at the photographs on pages 102 and 103. The same goes for the liver stir-fry. In the Fat meal the meat dominates. In Fit meals you can enjoy a good amount of meat and a lot more vegetables.

You may find that the sheer size of a 900 calorie meal made with whole, fresh food is too much for you. You don't have to eat it all, but part of the FAT TO FIT plan is that you fill yourself up with the right foods when you want to. If 900 calories is more than you can eat, you are probably a woman of average height, or shorter, with an average or small frame. 2,000 calories a day is about right for an 'average' woman. But of course there are many women who are in 'energy balance' at 1,800 or even 1,500 calories a day. A small, elderly woman who doesn't go out much will not want to eat much more than 1,500 calories a day, if that.

So if you find either of the Fit meals in this chapter are monsters, take smaller portions. Either cut back in proportion, or cut back rather more on the meat than the rice, potatoes, vegetables and fruit. After a while on the FAT TO FIT plan, once you have got used to hearty breakfasts, you may be inclined to eat much lighter suppers, so that your bigger meals are early in the day. If you prefer this pattern, it will be better for your digestion. In my grannie's day, 'dinner' was the midday meal, and 'tea', eaten as soon as the men got home from work at the end of the afternoon, was a cooked meal. Supper would be a small snack. These old-fashioned habits are uncommon now, except in families where the bread-winner goes to work very early in the morning. But they make a lot of sense.

If, like most people nowadays, you prefer to eat your main meal in the evening, that's fine. It's just a question of keeping to the basic principle of meals that are mostly whole, fresh cereals and vegetables. People in Britain and America, in particular, have got into the habit of thinking that a 'real meal' needs a slab of meat in the middle of the plate. This is bad news for health, and disaster for the

# WHAT'S SO SPECIAL ABOUT FIBRE

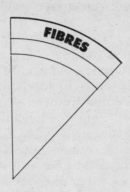

FIBRES

Before the Industrial Revolution, almost everybody, all over the world, ate plenty of fibre with their food. Without machines specially designed to strip it away and discard it, fibre was difficult to avoid.

Fibre forms the structure of all foods of vegetable origin. It's fibre that stands a plant up, like our skeletons. It's fibre that is wrapped round cereals, fruits, nuts, seeds and berries, as casing for their soft inner parts.

Until recently, most food contained fibre, but with industrialization everything changed. For example, fibre in whole sugar-cane and beet was stripped away in the 'refining' of processed white sugar. Likewise, most of the fibre in whole grain was lost in the making of white bread.

These mass-produced, cheap and uniform white sugars and white bread, drove out the healthy, relatively fibre-rich coarse breads.

Worse yet, until twenty or so years ago almost every nutritionist and food scientist agreed that fibre was useless as food. Laboratory tests seemed to show that fibre gave no energy to the body but just passed through. Many doctors believed that 'roughage' irritated the bowels and caused disease. 'Refined', highly processed food was, therefore just the stuff to give the troops.

As a result, the British food

slimmer. You have no need whatever to cut out meat. But think of it as an accompaniment to the meal, not as its centrepiece.

If you are vegetarian, that's fine too, of course, just as long as you kick out the saturated fats and processed sugars. Both the Fit suppers in this chapter are delicious without any meat at all.

By all means look through standard recipe books for

supply, in common with that of other Western and Westernized countries, is unnaturally short of fibre. It is estimated that average consumption of all types of fibre in Britain today is 18–20 grams per person per day. The target, to fill the Wheel of Health fibres segment, is 30 grams a day.

Just as vitamin B comes in different forms, there are different types of fibre with separate functions. Cereal fibre, from cereal sources such as wholegrains, peas and some other vegetables, is made of cellulose, which is not digested. This is why wholegrain bread is such an effective way to say goodbye to constipation forever.

There is now a great deal of reliable scientific evidence, provoked by the work of Dr Hugh Trowell and Dr Denis Burkitt, that indigestible (or 'insoluble') fibre, best eaten as part of whole cereal food, is vital to the good health of the entire gastro-intestinal tract.

The latest scientific news about fibre concerns 'soluble' fibres, the gums and pectins that are digestible in part. Oatmeal (as in porridge), beans, and the pips of fruit are rich in gums. Gums and pectins swell into gels in the gut (and are used as gelling agents by cooks and food manufacturers). Now you know why a big bowl of porridge is such a very satisfying breakfast: it's the gums in the oats that swell and keep you filled up.

While insoluble fibres nourish the gastro-intestinal tract, soluble fibres are now well-established as good for the cardiovascular system: they are good for the blood. Gums and pectins lower the level of harmful fats in the blood and protect against adult-onset diabetes. They may, therefore, also protect against heart attacks, although little laboratory work has yet been done to check out this reasonable assumption. So in the meantime the health message is: swallow it whole.

ideas for the family supper. Just about the only type of cooking to kick out of the window is French *haute cuisine*, which is stuffed with fats and sugars. Look for cook books from countries that have preserved a peasant tradition, like the countries all round the Mediterranean coastline, or India, or China. But a word of warning! Many cooks have mangled authentic recipes for the British market (as have many restaurant owners). Bring the balance back again by cutting out the fats and sugars and using lots more cereals and vegetables than the Westernized recipes suggest.

And there are plenty of good old-fashioned British suppers that can be part of the FAT TO FIT plan. How about a great plate of stew, for example? Improvise! My last stew was made of all the potatoes, tomatoes and green peppers left in the kitchen, together with onions and mushrooms lightly pre-fried in a little olive oil, plus tomato paste, a sprinkling of whole black peppercorns, simmered for an hour, and served with a new-fangled touch: yoghurt, borscht-style. It was good hot, and it was good cold the next day, too●

# RECOVERING OUR LOST ENERGY

Here is a remarkable fact. The total amount of energy, used for all her day's activities by a typical woman in Britain today, amounts to two ounces of roasted salted peanuts. Let me explain.

The body of a woman at complete rest, sleeping, or awake but not moving, uses just about exactly one calorie a minute. This 'Basal Metabolic Rate' (or BMR for short), therefore amounts to sixty calories an hour and 1,440 calories a day. Everybody is different of course, and metabolic rates vary, but whenever an average sort of woman leading an average sort of life has her BMR measured by scientists, it works out at around one calorie a minute.

Scientists have also worked out that the amount of calories women use up in total during a twenty-four hour day nowadays is around 2,000. This means that a woman will be in 'energy balance', neither gaining nor losing weight, when she consumes around 2,000 calories a day from food (and drink).

Roughly one tenth of the calories in food are 'lost' in extra heat generated by the body; this is known as 'Specific Dynamic Action' or SDA. It is now possible to do a rather fascinating sum, which goes as follows. BMR amounts to 1,440 calories a day; of 2,000 calories consumed, SDA amounts to 200 calories

# THE VALUE OF ACTIVITY

This table shows the energy value of twenty different activities and sports, per minute and per hour, measured in calories. The left hand column applies to women, the right hand column to men. The figures are of course approximations and some show a range of values depending on the vigour of the activity. Values will be higher for people who take regular exercise, because their metabolic rate is higher at all times.

| Activity | Women calories per | | Men calories per | |
| --- | --- | --- | --- | --- |
| | minute | hour | minute | hour |
| Sleeping | 1.0 | 60 | 1.3 | 78 |
| Resting | 1.1 | 66 | 1.4 | 84 |
| Sitting | 1.2 | 72 | 1.5 | 90 |
| Eating | 1.3 | 78 | 1.7 | 102 |
| Standing | 1.4 | 84 | 1.8 | 108 |
| Writing | 1.5 | 90 | 2.0 | 120 |
| Driving* | 2.0 | 120 | 2.5 | 150 |
| Mending | 2.0 | 120 | 2.5 | 150 |
| Cooking | 2.5 | 150 | 3.0 | 180 |
| Love-making* | 2.5–5.0 | 150–300 | 3.5–7.0 | 180–420 |
| Shopping | 3.0–4.0 | 180–240 | 4.0–6.0 | 240–360 |
| Walking | 3.0–5.0 | 180–300 | 4.0–7.0 | 240–420 |
| Cleaning | 3.0–6.0 | 180–360 | 4.0–8.0 | 240–480 |
| Gardening | 3.0–6.0 | 180–360 | 4.0–8.0 | 240–480 |
| Dancing | 3.0–6.0 | 180–360 | 4.0–8.0 | 240–480 |
| Tennis* | 3.0–6.0 | 180–360 | 4.0–8.0 | 240–480 |
| Climbing | 4.0–7.0 | 240–420 | 5.0–9.0 | 300–540 |
| Swimming | 6.0–10.0 | 360–600 | 8.0–12.0 | 480–720 |
| Running | 6.0–12.0 | 360–720 | 8.0–16.0 | 480–960 |
| Squash* | 8.0–12.0 | 480–720 | 10.0–16.0 | 600–960 |

* when in motion

a day. Adding 1,440 and 200 together comes to 1,640. So it follows that any woman in energy balance at 2,000 calories a day uses a mere 360 calories a day for all her activity. Two ounces of peanuts contain 360 calories.

If you've ever 'been on a diet', you will know that the main idea is to decrease the amount of energy (calories) you consume from food and drink, without changing your level of activity (some books nowadays recommend exercise, but they are usually rather vague). In other words you under-feed yourself, paying careful attention to the energy (calorie) value of food, but without paying any special attention to the value of activity.

The FAT TO FIT plan works because it operates the other way round. The idea is that you transform the quality of the food you consume while keeping up its quantity (measured in terms of energy value). **Do not cut calories.** Do not semi-starve yourself. Instead, pay careful attention to your activity and its energy value, and increase the amount of energy you use in activity above its present level, to the value of 300 calories a day for a woman, 400 calories a day for a man – see pages 45–48.

Now look at the chart 'The Value of Activity', on page 61. The figures on the left show the energy (calorie) values of twenty different common forms of activity and exercise for a typical woman; those on the right apply to a typical man. Everybody is different and the exact energy value of any activity varies, of course, with the individual, but not that greatly. The main difference is that anybody who is lean will use more energy all the time because lean tissue and muscle are designed to be more metabolically active.

Our problem, and the key reason why we are liable to get fat while eating less and less food, is that we spend too much time on the activities in the top half of the table and not enough time on the activities in the bottom half. It is literally true that apart from an occasional dash for the bus, the most energetic activity for millions of people nowadays is making love, which is no doubt why so many people are rotten love-makers. They just can't keep going.

As you can see, most of the activities in the top half of the table have a fixed energy value. Sleeping, after all, is sleeping; most people do not wave their arms about or walk in their sleep. The value of some of these activities will vary a bit, depending on how you do them.

The value of the activities in the bottom half of the table can vary greatly. 'Cleaning', for example, can vary between polishing a table (three calories a minute) and scrubbing the floor (six calories a minute).

The values given are based on the assumption that you are actually active. Lying in bed only thinking about making love scores somewhere around 1.1 to 1.2. And you will not score much above mending or cooking if you lie back and only think about the FAT TO FIT plan. Once at it, the value will depend on style.

What you can do if you choose, starting today, is to put those missing 300 calories a day back into your life, just by walking. This extra 2,000 calories a week will make you fitter and healthier. It will also make you slimmer.

Work it out for yourself. If you eat the same amount of food as you eat now, but increase your activity by 2,000 calories a week, that amounts to the calorie value of just over half a pound of body fat. (Most books say that a pound of fat amounts to around 3,500 calories). Over a period of twenty-six weeks, that adds up to almost a stone of body weight. But, better than that, you will also find that after some time you will be gaining slim, lean tissue, while losing fat. The result is that you may not lose a great deal of weight during the six months of this plan, but you should lose a lot of fat, and be slimmer.

Back to walking. If you step out and actually get puffed, you will be using up maybe 240 calories an hour, which is 180 more than the resting (BMR) rate of 60 an hour. This means that if you choose to walk briskly for an extra 100 minutes a day, you would get those missing 300 calories a day back into your life.

That sounds like a lot of time. But is it? For example, suppose you work in an office, and your office is half an hour from home (on foot), and that the local shops are fifteen minutes away from the office. During the week, you could stop waiting for buses or other transport and walk for a total of ninety minutes instead. And if at the weekend you go for a two hour walk on Saturday and Sunday, that would all average 100 minutes a day●

# WHERE'S YOUR ACTION?

Have you ever stopped to think how active you are during an average day? Here's your chance to work it out. Listed below are ten common forms of activity and exercise. Rate your own activity on a typical weekday by putting a tick in the box that applies to you. There are two extra rows in which to insert any regular activity or exercise of yours not already listed.

If your level of activity varies from day to day (for example, because you go to exercise classes, or take long walks at weekends, or whatever) and if you have access to a copying machine, take extra copies of this page. Or you might prefer to fill in your average level of activity over a whole week, rather than a day – whatever suits you best.

First, though, rate your *level* of activity. Think of other people you know; family, friends, or at work. Do you reckon you are more active than they are? Less active? Or would you say you are about average? We'll be asking again later in the plan.

Compared with other people I know, I would say I am

| Very active | Average | Inactive |
|---|---|---|
| | | |

On an average sort of day the amount of time I take in activity is

| Minutes | none | 1–10 | 10–30 | 30–60 | 60 plus |
|---|---|---|---|---|---|
| Cooking | | | | | |
| Cycling | | | | | |
| Dancing | | | | | |
| Driving | | | | | |
| Gardening | | | | | |
| Housework | | | | | |
| Running | | | | | |
| Shopping | | | | | |
| Swimming | | | | | |
| Walking | | | | | |
| Other (name) | | | | | |
| Other (name) | | | | | |

# FAT to FIT

## 4

# HAVE A GOOD LUNCH

**V**egetables? I can hear you now: 'Boring. Besides, fresh vegetables may be good for slimmers, and may be healthy: but what a fag to prepare!' ● If you are at home for lunch, this chapter is for you. Just see the difference between processed and real home-made soup, and find out how easy good soup is to make ● And yes, tinned food can be Fit food, if you know which tins to choose ● How to go from Fat to Fit if you have a small appetite, or if you are elderly ● Advice on vitamin pills ● How housework needn't be a chore and can help you lose weight

You're at home in the morning, and you're wondering what to have for lunch. Maybe you're by yourself; maybe you're with your children; maybe it's the weekend. In any case, you fancy something tasty. I work at home, and round about mid-day I start to feel like a little something. And that's the point at which I have a roam around the kitchen to see what's on offer. 'This won't do any harm' you think to yourself, picking up an item. 'This'll do'. And if you feel a bit tired or rushed, or want to keep the kids quiet, you'll feel inclined to rustle up something quick.

Soup, for instance. You will have seen advertisements

for tinned or packet soup, on television and in the shops. Happy, smiling, glowing people sipping nectar? Or else thatched cottages, roses round the door, kitchen interior with olde Welsh dresser, dimpled grannie with a ladle-full of amber liquid.

And why do you have tinned or packaged soup in your larder? Because it's cheap, because it's simple, and because soup has a nice homely, comforting image. Correct? Besides (you think as you're walking past the rows and rows of processed soups in the supermarket), soup can't do me any harm. It won't make me fat . . .

What do the labels of popular, packaged soups look like? Brace yourself:

Ingredients: Modified wheat starch, glucose syrup, salt; flavour enhancers, monosodium glutamate, sodium 5-ribonucleotide; dextrose, vegetable fat, tomato powder, hydrolysed vegetable protein, yeast extract, dried onion, onion powder, spices, flavouring; colours E150, E123, E102; caseinate, acidity regulator E340; emulsifiers E471, E472 (b); antioxidant E320.

That was 'onion' 'soup'. This next one is 'celery' 'soup':

Ingredients: maltodextrin, vegetable fat, modified starch, salt, flavourings including celery, dried celery; flavour enhancer, monosodium glutamate; onion powder, gelling agent E415, dried parsley; colour E102, E110, brilliant blue FCF.

And the third marvel of modern food science is old-fashioned, tinned vegetable soup:

Ingredients: carrots, potatoes, onions, peas, green beans, leeks, tomato purée, sugar, modified starch, salt, haricot beans, flour, vegetable oil, pearl barley, hydrolysed vegetable protein; flavour enhancer, monosodium glutamate; spices, herbs.

The mysterious world of chemical additives is explained in

# THE CHOICE IS YOURS

## LUNCH AT HOME

| | FAT<br>600 calories | FIT (1)<br>600 calories | FIT (2)<br>600 calories |
|---|---|---|---|
| | Vegetable soup (dried, packet) (7 oz) | Vegetable soup (home-made): carrots (4 oz), leeks (4 oz), parsnip (4 oz), tomato (4 oz), parsley; butter (¼ oz) | Salad: crab (tinned) (3½ oz), kidney beans (tinned) (3½ oz); sweetcorn (tinned) (3½ oz), cucumber (4 oz); mustard and cress (4 oz); dressing (oil and lemon) (1 tbsp) |
| | Cheese on toast (one thick slice) (3½ oz) | Bread (one slice, wholemeal) Jacket potato (7 oz) filled with mushrooms (4 oz), onion (4 oz), oil (1½ tsp) | Wholemeal roll (2½ oz) |
| | Sponge cake with jam (2½ oz) | Grapes (5 oz) | Cherries (4 oz) |
| Saturated fats | HEAVY | LIGHT | LIGHT |
| Sugars | HEAVY | LIGHT | LIGHT |
| Salt | HEAVY | LIGHT** | LIGHT** |
| Additives | HEAVY | LIGHT | LIGHT |
| Proteins | RICH | RICH | SUPER-RICH |
| Starches | POOR | MEDIUM | MEDIUM |
| Fibres | POOR | SUPER-RICH | SUPER-RICH |
| Essential fats | POOR | RICH | RICH |
| Vitamin $B_6$ | POOR | RICH | RICH |
| Folic acid (Fo) | POOR | RICH | SUPER-RICH |
| Potassium (K) | POOR | SUPER-RICH | RICH |
| Iron (Fe) | POOR | RICH | RICH |

** if not added

Key to terms used here and on Wheels of Health: page 199.
Fit soup and salad recipes: Chapter 9.

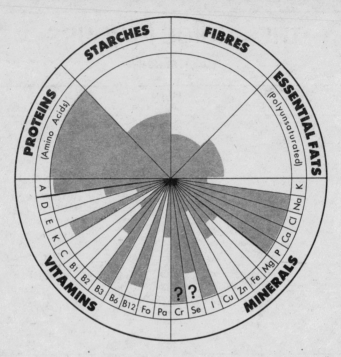

● **Fat lunch: processed soup, cheese on toast, cake.** It's quick, it's easy, it's cheap, and it's nasty. The slug of salt in the soup will make you thirsty and un-satisfied. The fatty cheese and the fatty and sugary cake leave empty spaces in your stomach and also in the Wheel. If you (and your family) regularly eat 'convenience food' like this you'll be short-changed for nourishment and you'll end up fat. (Menu: page 67.)

other books. That aside, notice that the three soups contain four helpings of added sugars (glucose syrup, dextrose, maltodextrin and sugar); three of added fats; and no less than six pourings of salt (including three sodium compounds).

This is a far cry from the soup that grannie used to make, with or without rosy dimples. Do you really want to feed yourself or your family with processed fats, sugars

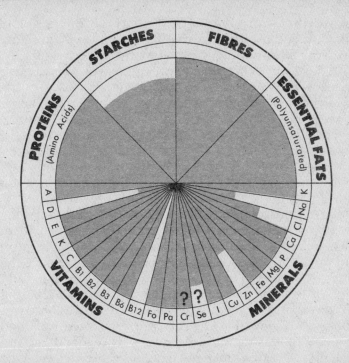

● **Fit lunch: home-made soup, bread, jacket potato, fruit.** 'Go on! Fill 'em up with soup like mother used to make' say the ads. It's good advice, when you cook genuine home-made soup. Yes, this soup, and the baked potato, does take some preparation, but how highly do you value your health? This is a super meal for kids: 600 calories, same as the Fat lunch, but very satisfying. (Menu: page 67. Recipe: page 164.)

---

and salt? If you have kids, ask them to read out the label of 'onion' 'soup', that I've just listed, and ask them what they think. Will they say 'yummy yummy' or 'ugh'?

Of course, you are not going to keel over as a result of eating one, or a dozen, packets of chemicalized soup. But incessant eating of products to which fats, sugars and salt are added, is almost certain to harm your health in some way. Certainly, fats and sugars make you fat; directly, because they are concentrated slugs of calories, and indirectly because they don't fill you up, and therefore leave you feeling hungry. So after the hi-tech soup you might have some cheese on toast, and maybe a small piece of packet cake. More fats, sugars and salt.

Real home-made soup takes time to prepare. There's the shopping for the vegetables, the peeling and cutting, the checking with a recipe book, the simmering, the draining, the serving . . . Do you resent the idea of all this housework? If you do, sit back and think about how you spend your day. In particular, think about the things you enjoy doing.

Food manufacturers believe that more than anything else we want cheap food. The result is cheapened food, which nobody values much at any price. We have been conditioned to think of food as fuel and – if we have the money – as a feast. Unlike people in France, Germany and Italy, for example, we have lost the pleasure of preparing everyday food at home. It's become drudgery, 'a chore'.

Once you know that the difference between bad food and good food is the difference between Fat and Fit, and much more besides, you'll put a higher value on food. One of the pleasures I remember as a child was coming home and, even before the front door opened, smelling soup simmering. It's that sense of warmth and welcome that makers of packaged soup play on, in their advertising. But when I was a child, it wasn't dried glucose syrup or mono-sodium glutamate I was smelling, but the real thing: fresh vegetables. 'Oh, it's all very well for Geoffrey Cannon writing this nostalgia about home-made soup' (do I hear you think?). 'When he was a child it wasn't him doing the cooking.' Yes, I agree that many people, parents especially, have their hands full at home. Yes, it's true that I don't spend all my days stirring cauldrons of goodies, either. And yes, we can enjoy the advantages of con-venience food.

But convenient to whom? You, or the food industry?

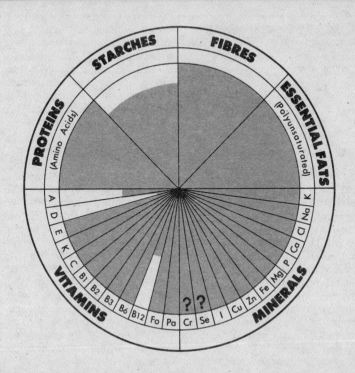

● **Fit lunch: crab and bean salad, bread, fruit.** It's quick, it's easy, and it's very good for you. Some tinned food is fine when you know what to choose. This crab salad is a summer treat: cheaper alternatives are tuna or sardine. It's 600 calories again, an almost perfectly balanced meal as you can see from the Wheel. It's also super-rich in many nutrients. (Menu: page 67. Recipe without the crab: page 162.)

Let's replay the beginning of this chapter. You're at home in the morning and you're wondering what to have for lunch. You have a roam around the kitchen to see what's on offer. But this time, because you've started to read food labels, there are no chemicalized nectars on your shelves. Instead, you have a stack of fresh vegetables.

Do you have to spend the best part of an hour preparing soup? No, you don't. Firstly, if you have a blender, home-

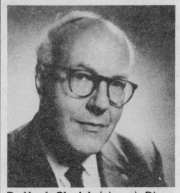

**Dr Hugh Sinclair** (above), Director of the International Institute of Human Nutrition in Oxford, is the living British nutritionist who above all, perhaps, can be called a genius. As a young man in the 1930s he became convinced of the fundamental importance of good food, to preserve health and to protect against disease.

'Flour, with bread made from it, is the most important single item in our diets', maintains Dr Sinclair. So he has always fought for high quality, especially wholegrain, flour and bread. Thirty years ago he sounded an alarm about white bread, which has most of the goodness in the whole grain processed out of it. Of vitamin $B_6$ and folic acid, lost in white bread, Dr Sinclair wrote that they 'are grossly neglected, interact with each other and are, I believe, very important in human nutrition.'

He has always spoken his mind, and so has made people in government and industry uncomfortable. For instance, a few vitamins are partially restored, by the industry, to white bread. What does he think of that? He replies by quoting from Dorothy L Sayers' thriller *Murder Must Advertise*: 'By forcing the damn-fool public to pay twice over – once to have its food emasculated and once to have the vitality put in again, we keep the wheels of commerce turning'.

The official Department of Health view is that the British people are well fed – if anything, too well fed. Dr Sinclair has always seen things quite differently. In his view Western food is impoverished.

made soup becomes a convenience food. Second, you don't have to make soup. My son Ben was quite a star cook at university, specializing in making fast, fresh-food meals from cheap ingredients. One of his favourites, and mine, is what he calls 'Anything Goes In Stew', which is self-explanatory. Give the vegetables that come to hand a scrub, slice them, bung them in a pot with water, without salt but with herbs, and leave to simmer. Vegetable stew is helped by a little olive oil, and a small tin of tomato purée. Certain vegetables, like onions, are best fried first, but that only takes a couple of minutes. 'Anything Goes In Stew' can of course include little tasty bits of meat: bacon, for instance, fried first with the onions, or left-over chicken.

If by any chance you don't eat all of your 'Anything Goes In Stew' at one sitting, you'll find it tastes even better the next day, when the flavours will have mingled. Reheat it gently, and if you want to stretch it even further, add some more chopped-up fresh vegetables and herbs.

What you do need, for good stews, is thick, heavy cast-iron pots that distribute heat efficiently. They are expensive but save on heat. Thin metal pots are no good for stews. And don't use aluminium: it's a toxic metal.

Am I saying that you should never eat tinned food? No. After all, I've already recommended tomato purée. Tinned whole tomatoes are a versatile good buy, for example. But check all tins for added salt or sugar. And there are a number of vegetables that come in very handy for summer salad lunches. Beans, for example, and sweetcorn, are good supermarket choices for a quick meal. They're cooked in the tin; all you have to do is turn them out and make them extra delicious with fresh salads like cucumber and tomato, and with a generous brushing of lemon and olive oil dressing, plus garlic if you like.

Some tinned fish is a good standby, too. Tuna and sardines are tasty: be prepared to spend a little more on fish packed in olive oil or in water. For a treat open a tin of crab with your salad. Always drain tinned food before use.

Most of the meals devised for FAT TO FIT add up to 2000 calories a day. This is because it's reliably reckoned that the 'average' woman in Western countries today who is in 'energy balance', neither gaining nor losing weight, is eating around 2000 calories of energy a day, from food.

# THE VITAL A B C (and D E)

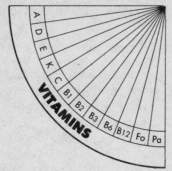

We've all heard of vitamins A, B, C and D. These were the first to be identified as vital to life (hence the name 'vita-min', and the alphabetical order). Half a century ago, vitamins were big news. Scientists had isolated a few of them and found that food drained of specific vitamins caused 'deficiency' diseases, such as scurvy (gross deficiency of vitamin C), rickets (vitamin D, also created by the body from sunlight), and beri-beri (vitamin $B_1$). In the 1930s, people in government and science insisted that food manufacturers maintained standard levels of officially 'scheduled' vitamins in staple foods. Hence the vitamins A and D added to margarine, the vitamins $B_1$ and $B_3$ added to white flour and thence bread, and fruit syrups and drinks advertised as rich in vitamin C.

**V**itamins are a Good Thing, because they are Good For You. Everybody knows that. Vitamins are potent and mysterious little fellows. They're there, but you can't see them. They are synthesized and sold as pills in 'health food' shops, so they seem to be some sort of remedy.

But why do they matter? Doesn't a 'normal, balanced, varied diet' contain enough vitamins? Besides, what have vitamins got to do with losing excess fat?

An early name for vitamins was 'protective factors'. When government was keen to protect the health of the popula-

The figure for the 'average' man is around 2600 calories a day. Therefore, if you are average, and transform the quality of your food, and increase the quantity of your activity, you will lose fat on 2000 calories of food a day.

If 2000 calories is too much for you, you will soon find out. This is because whole food is bulky: it fills you up literally, physically. Feeling full is fine; for calorie-cutting slimmers, it's one of life's lost pleasures, and of course FAT

tion, whose welfare used to be seen as a national asset, great efforts were made to promote foods rich in vitamins. Official public health messages explained why we all need vitamins A, B, C and D for good health, together with protein, calcium (Ca) and iron (Fe). These are the nutrients still 'scheduled' by the Department of Health.

But vitamins protect not only negatively, against disease, but also positively; for good health. For instance, various vitamins in the B complex are vital to the nervous system. Long before any sign of beriberi diagnosable by a doctor, lack of $B_1$ (and other vitamins) is a cause of fatigue, inertia and depression. So foods rich in B vitamins are a crucial means to progress from Fat to Fit.

A great deal is now known about the function of vitamins, including others included in the Wheel of Health which are still not officially 'scheduled' by the Department of Health – E, K, $B_6$, $B_{12}$, folic acid (Fo) and panthothenic acid (Pa). For example, foods rich in vitamins A, C and E are likely to protect against various cancers. Birth defects are probably caused in part by a diet poor in folic acid (and other nutrients). Vitamin $B_6$ is often called 'the woman's vitamin' because shortage may provoke menstrual disorders.

If you eat food rich in the vitamins shown on the Wheel of Health, you will be eating a genuinely balanced diet. People who eat lots of whole, fresh food are unlikely to be short of vitamins (or any other nutrients) unless they abuse their bodies with tobacco, alcohol or drugs. The fact is that the British food supply is abnormal, unbalanced and short of vitamins. Official recommendations for animal vitamin intakes used by farmers, animal breeders and zoo keepers are higher – sometimes much higher – than levels contained in the human food supply.

**Note:** for an explanation of the standards for vitamins used in the Wheels, see reference 19 on page 186.

TO FIT is designed to encourage you to regain that pleasure.

But if the result of a 700 calorie lunch, say, or a 900 calorie supper, is to make you feel full and sleepy, then the meal may well be more than you need. In that case all you need to do is follow the plan, but cut down the amount you eat, in proportion. Two words of caution, though. First, please don't reduce the amount you eat at breakfast. The heartier your first meal of the day the better.

# VITAMIN PILLS

Eat good food, not bad food plus pills. That's the first advice to give to anybody thinking of spending their money on vitamin pills. The best place to find vitamins, and all other nutrients, is in whole fresh food where nature put them. Everybody knows that oranges are rich in vitamin C. It's a pity that shops don't promote potatoes as rich in vitamin C too; or that it's A for apricots, B complex for bread, and so on.

Vitamin and mineral pills can be expensive. And the mark-up between manufacturer and the retail shop is often outrageous.

Cost aside, there are two big worries about pills. First, many of the people behind the counter in shops that sell vitamin and mineral pills don't know much about them. And second, vitamins and minerals come in balanced packages, in nature, but not in the shops. SuperThis is stacked next to MegaThat and Ultimate The Other. If *you* don't know what it all means, and the shop assistant doesn't know either, why buy?

Companies selling their vitamin or mineral pill formulation often imply that you can't have too much of a good thing. This is simply not true. Gross overdoses of fat-soluble vitamins A, D, E and K can be poisonous (not, though, in the amounts found in any individual pill). Also, megadoses of any vitamin – and strong doses of any mineral – throw the body's absorption of these nutrients out of balance. And in the long run that can be dangerous.

Adolescents, women thinking of becoming pregnant, and old people, *may* need multivitamin and mineral pills; and anybody who has suffered shock will certainly need supplements. Other people can benefit from nutritional therapy with professional guidance.

Oh yes: there is no such thing as a vitamin pill that makes you slim. Just stick to good food.

Second, watch your snacking. If you feel uncomfortably full after a good meal, but also pack in a couple of chocolate biscuits or a confectionery bar on the side, it's not the Fit meals you should cut down on. Craving for chemicalized sweet fat is a problem. If you feel addicted to sugars and sugary fats, I'm not going to pretend that you'll be cured after a day or a week of Fit food. It takes longer than that. FAT TO FIT isn't magic●

# WHISTLE WHILE YOU HOUSEWORK

In 1985, a team of scientists working in Cambridge announced some new discoveries about the value of everyday activity. These overturn all the conventional wisdom about the effect modern living has on our health and fitness, and show yet again why calorie counting is wrong.

For many years now, it's been officially agreed that the 'average' adult woman needs and uses around 2200 calories of energy from food, every day. The official figure for men is just under 3000 calories. These figures are based on the assumption that for every ten calories women use for the unconscious activity of the body, they need and use another five calories for their own conscious everyday activity. The body's own activity, including the work of the liver, brain, heart and digestive system, is called 'basal metabolic rate' or BMR for short. Therefore official figures are based on the assumption that the average woman is in 'energy balance', neither gaining nor losing weight, at BMR plus seventy per cent, or 1.7 BMR.

Only when women are over fifty-five, 'assuming a sedentary life', do the official figures approach 2000 calories a day. And the experts have supposed that an 'average' woman needs to be over seventy-five years old before her energy balance is under 2000 calories a day.

Using brand new techniques, however, Dr Andrew Prentice, Dr Andrew Coward, and colleagues at the Dunn Clinical Nutrition Centre, have proved beyond reasonable doubt that the official figures are way out. They are too high – for many people, far too high. The truth is that for every ten calories of unconscious activity (BMR), an average woman now uses only three to four extra calories in conscious activity. That is to say, we are only half as active as the official figures suggest.

Even more disturbing, young women nowadays typically need and use only 2000 calories a day from food, or even less. This means that a woman aged thirty in 1986 is likely

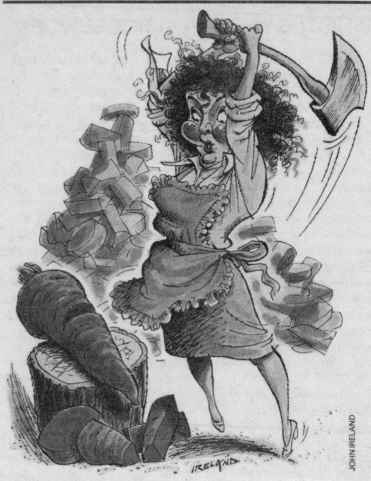

JOHN IRELAND

to be no more active than a woman of sixty was, only thirty years ago. Some young women nowadays are in energy balance at 1800 calories a day, or even lower. The amount of energy they use is not much more than that of an infirm old lady who sits in a chair all day. Such people are likely to lead pretty miserable lives, gaining fat if they eat the same amount of food as their family and friends, finding it impossible to lose weight unless they starve themselves, and at risk from diseases caused by chronic lack of nourishment.

Why? In the 1940s and 1950s, the official figures may well have been correct. But now they do not take into account the effect of the everyday use of machines. Everybody makes use of electricity, gas and petrol. 'Laboursaving' machines do the work our bodies are designed to do. Dr Prentice agrees that it is vital for health and fitness to become active; to take the 'average' person, now more sedentary than ever before, to being twice as active.

'Housework' has a bad image. Men don't like housework because they feel it's woman's work. I remember once preparing a dinner party to be given jointly by me and my son Ben, who was hard at it shopping and preparing the vegetables. Ben's friend Dave came round to support. 'Is there anything I can do?' he asked. I was laying the table at the time. 'Thank you' I said. 'Yes, there is. Sweep the floor.' Pause. Long pause. He looked embarrassed. 'But' he said 'men don't sweep floors.'

Women don't like housework because they object to men not sharing the responsibility. So, given the opportunity, men avoid being active at home, and women insist on machines to do the work as compensation. Anything domestic involving muscles becomes a bore, a chore, a sign of inferior status.

One way to move from Fat to Fit, and to restore your lost energy, is to become more active at home. I am not saying that we should all install coppers and mangles and do the washing by hand. What I am suggesting is that you think about what activity in the house you actually rather enjoy, and choose to use your body more, at home. The questionnaire on page 80 is a means for you to assess your own level of activity at home: and on page 175 there's a plan for restoring that lost 300 calories a day●

# DAILY DOMESTIC DOZEN

Is your day at home all go? Or have machines taken your life over? Do you do the shopping and the cooking, the dusting and the ironing? Do you spend your day leaping around with babies or children? Or sitting in an armchair?

Below is listed a range of domestic activities, plus a couple of rows for you to fill in any activity of yours not in the list. If you have babies or children, there's space for them too. The idea this time is not only to rate the frequency of your domestic activity, but also how you feel about it. So don't just tick the boxes. Write 'Love', 'Like', 'OK', 'Dislike' or 'Hate' instead. For example, if you make beds every day and hate it, write 'Hate' in the left hand column. First, though, rate your overall level of activity compared with others'.

Compared with other people I know, I would say I am

| Very active | Average | Inactive |
|---|---|---|
| | | |

I would rate the level of my activity at home, and how I feel about it, as follows:

| | Daily | Every other day | Weekly | Monthly | Never |
|---|---|---|---|---|---|
| Bed-making | | | | | |
| Carpentry | | | | | |
| Cleaning* | | | | | |
| Cooking | | | | | |
| Decorating | | | | | |
| Other DIY | | | | | |
| Dusting | | | | | |
| Ironing | | | | | |
| Laundry | | | | | |
| Vacuum cleaning | | | | | |
| Washing-up | | | | | |
| Window cleaning | | | | | |
| Other (name) | | | | | |
| Other (name) | | | | | |
| Babies | | | | | |
| Children | | | | | |

# FAT TO FIT

## 5

# LITTLE SOMETHINGS

**S**nack food and fast food is booming in Britain. For many people, particularly the young, 'proper' sit-down meals have almost become a thing of the past ● How to tell the difference between snacks that make you Fat and snacks that make you Fit ● Elemental health: the need for minerals, and new ways to guard against eating disorders like 'anorexia nervosa' ● The politics of food: why you are not getting the full story about the foods that make you Fat ● And the secrets revealed about calorie-cutting diets and the dieting industry

How many times do you eat, every day? Once upon a time (or so it's supposed) we all sat down with our families, three times a day, for Square Meals. Now, though, cooked breakfasts and meat-and-two-veg are endangered species, to be seen in railway dining-cars, restaurants, hotels and at weekends, but only occasionally in everyday homes. We have taken to eating food 'on the hoof', or to 'grazing': meals are being replaced by snacks.

In America, two industries are booming above all others: hi-tech food and hi-tech 'health care'. The big bucks are in fast food and fat farms. Shrewd investors are putting their money into hamburger franchises and heart bypass units; irradiation of fruit and transplantation of vital organs; extrusion technology and micro-slimming clubs. For processed food manufacturers, a new chemical flavour is flavour of the month. We are into space-age food. But how do we avoid major malfunction?

My advice is to develop a healthy cynicism about claims made by the snack manufacturers. Sir Douglas Black, a wise man who in his time as president of the Royal College of Physicians presided over a key report on obesity, once remarked 'if something has to be advertised, there's probably something wrong with it'. Certainly, as a rule, the more a food is advertised the worse it is likely to be for your health.

Close your eyes and bring to mind every snack you have ever eaten. Of the scores – maybe hundreds – of choices, which snack food is so cleverly packaged that you can pick it straight up and put it in your bag or pocket or office drawer, in all weathers, and eat it half a day later, just as fresh as it was when you first fancied it?

That's an easy question to answer. Fruit, of course. Apples and oranges are available all the year round, but are often pretty tasteless in the summer. Be adventurous. Make a detour to your local street market, or find a greengrocer with imagination. Apricots and peaches are super-rich in vitamin A. Pounce on plums and damsons in season. Keep a knife and spoon in the office, and share a melon or a couple of mangoes with friends. Snap up strawberries, raspberries, blackberries, redcurrants, blackcurrants and other soft fruit when they're fully ripe, and eat them as they come.

There's a simple rule with fruit. You can't eat too much of it. All fruit is rich in potassium (K), and much fruit is a good source of magnesium (Mg) – two minerals that most people are short of (see the Wheel of Health for the national food supply on page 97). Fruit is beautiful; buy big bowls and arrange fruit in them, and make fruit a centrepiece at table. If you've got children, be pleased when they stuff an orange or a banana into their pocket or mouth as they walk through a room or off to school. It's worth knowing, too, that while

# THE CHOICE IS YOURS

## SNACKS

| | FAT (1) 250 calories | FAT (2) 250 calories | FIT (1) 250 calories | FIT (2) 250 calories |
|---|---|---|---|---|
| | Doughnut (1½oz) Cola drink (11.6floz) | Biscuits (2–3 chocolate digestives, 2oz) | Bread (1 slice) Camembert cheese (1½oz) Celery (2 sticks) Fruit (apricots, 7½oz) | Yoghurt (5oz) Raisins (1oz) Oatmeal (¾oz) |
| Saturated fats | HEAVY | HEAVY | MEDIUM | LIGHT |
| Sugars | HEAVY | HEAVY | LIGHT | LIGHT |
| Salt | LIGHT | MEDIUM | HEAVY | LIGHT |
| Additives | HEAVY | MEDIUM* | LIGHT | LIGHT |
| Proteins | POOR | POOR | SUPER-RICH | SUPER-RICH |
| Starches | POOR | POOR | POOR | POOR |
| Fibres | POOR | POOR | RICH | RICH |
| Essential fats | POOR | POOR | POOR | POOR |
| Vitamin B₁ | POOR | POOR | RICH | RICH |
| Vitamin C | POOR** | POOR** | RICH | POOR |
| Calcium (Ca) | POOR | POOR | SUPER-RICH | SUPER-RICH |
| Zinc (Zn) | POOR | POOR | RICH | RICH |

* depending on recipe    ** actually, empty
Key to terms used here and on Wheels of Health: page 199.
Fit snack ideas: Chapter 9.

fruit can be expensive, if you eat more wholegrain bread, cereal products and vegetables, and less meat, your weekly shopping bill can balance.

Nature's other ingeniously packaged snack food is, of course, nuts. Buy nuts whole and keep them fresh. The ritual of cracking nuts also slows down the rate at which you eat them. All fresh nuts are super-rich in essential fats and a number of minerals and trace elements. They are also very

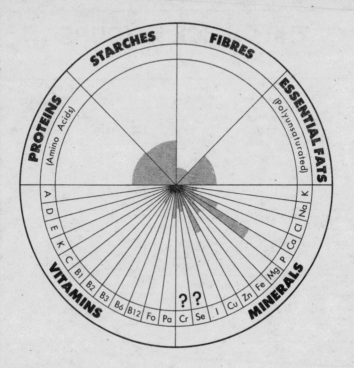

● **Fat snack: doughnut and cola drink.** When you put 'fun foods' on the Wheel, they don't look such fun any more. Processed, 'refined' sugars, and saturated fats supply nothing but calories: their Wheels are totally empty. A couple of bites of a doughnut (1½ ounces) and a can of cola drink contain 250 calories – one eighth of a daily 2,000 calorie requirement – and that's just about all.

concentrated sources of calories: lay off the shelled peanuts and cashew nuts which are also drenched in salt.

Commercial snack food is mostly dead food. Products with a long shelf life are made with saturated fats and processed sugars or salt, because these are good commodities: they don't 'go off', which is because there's nothing in them to nourish rodents, insects or micro-organisms. So they're served up to you instead. Look at the 'menu' for the Fat

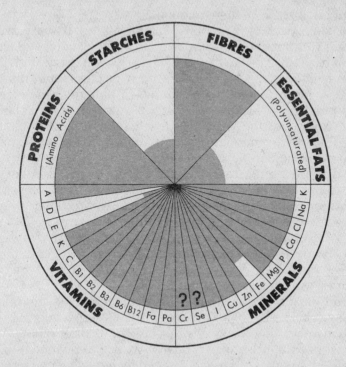

● **Fit snack: bread and cheese, celery and fruit.** You can't expect any snack to be full of all the nourishment you need. But this simple snack, also providing 250 calories, is super-rich in a number of vitamins and minerals. Good bread and cheese is best without butter, as here. Followed by almost half a pound of fruit, this is as good as a light meal. (Menu: page 83.)

snacks on page 83, and you will see that they are all poor sources of proteins, starches, fibres, essential fats, and virtually every vitamin and mineral.

At home, a slice of good, fresh, wholegrain bread, and cheese, together with fruit, is a Fit snack, balanced just about as well as fruit and nuts. If you have a blender at home, try mixes of fruits together with yoghurt, plus some whole grains, like oats, to give the mixture some body – not to mention fibres, B vitamins and minerals.

Become your own fast food manufacturer. If there are kids in your family, do invest in a juicer and blender, and let them have fun making cocktails of snacks with every kind of colour, flavour and texture. Mix up fruit purées and thick juices from the whole fruit, with bits of pith and skin, core and pip, and drink the result as a pick-me-up at breakfast time. Show kids the Wheel of Health and get them to fill it in, using their own mixtures of Fit foods from the ideas and recipes in Chapter nine.

Advertisers often call Fat food 'fun food', because that's just about the only legal claim that can be made for it. Consumption of biscuits and chocolate confectionery, in Britain, is the highest in the world. And as you can see from the Wheels opposite, these are grossly Fat foods. Two and a half chocolate digestives pack in 250 calories. If you keep the packet open and eat five, that's a quarter of your daily calories, with virtually no nourishment.

And sugar and sweets? The Wheel of Health for sugars is empty. That's why sugars are rightly called 'empty calories'.

Remember that hunger is not just for calories (energy). We all need nourishment – quality, as well as quantity – in our food. At times of growth we need high-quality food even more, and plenty of it. Babies, young children, adolescents and pregnant women are hungry for vitamins and minerals, as well as energy. In pregnancy, women often crave strange foods, and may even eat things like coal. Little children often eat dirt. Doctors who know nothing about nutrition think such behaviour is bizarre, but it's normal. Animals search out the nutrients their bodies need and, when they are ill, will move away from their usual eating places to find plants and soil rich in special vitamins and minerals.

And here is a key reason why people in Western countries so often become fat. Food loaded with fats and sugars is drained of nourishment. Therefore, it is not satisfying. The human animal, 'on the hoof', snacking on Fat food, is in effect continually roaming around seeking a sense of satis-

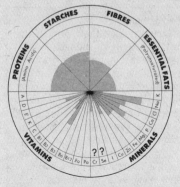

● **Fat snack: chocolate digestive biscuits.** Any goodness in it is swamped by fats and sugars.

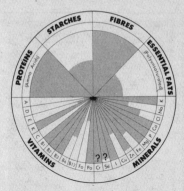

● **Fit snack: yoghurt, raisins, oatmeal.** Here's a muesli bar without the fatty, sugary binding.

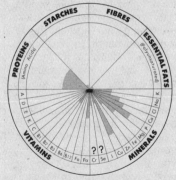

● **Fat snack: chocolate bar.** A great slug of worthless empty calories, made from sugar and fats.

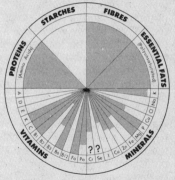

● **Fit snack: fruit and nuts.** This combination is an example of nature's own fast food.

faction, and never finding it. Some people believe that 'junk' or 'trash' food is a cause of anti-social, even violent behaviour. It is certainly true that chemical dyes and some preservatives used in highly-processed foods send many children 'up the wall'. Anybody who continually eats food drained of B vitamins and minerals will become depressed and lethargic and suffer from 'mood swings'. The true fun food is Fit food. After all, everybody knows that pets need

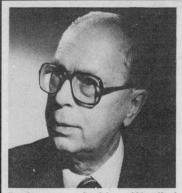

**Professor Arvid Wretlind** (above) of the Karolinska Institute in Stockholm, is a nutritionist and also a statesman. Over twenty years ago, in the mid-1960s, he realized that the Western food supply, as eaten in Britain, America (and Sweden), was a major threat to public health.

The problem, as he saw it, was – and still is – that in the last hundred years, staple starchy foods, bread and potatoes in particular, have been replaced by fatty and sugary items. The result is a pattern of diseases: tooth decay, constipation, brittle bones, anaemia, heart disease, and obesity.

Having identified the problem, he then proposed a solution, in an action programme presented to the Swedish government. Since then, over fifty national 'dietary goals' reports have been produced all over the Western world. Arvid Wretlind was first. What everybody needs for good health, he said, is more cereal foods, green and root vegetables and fruit; and much fewer fats and sugars.

He was also the first to realize the dangers for inactive people. The less you eat, the more nourishing or 'nutrient-dense' your food needs to be. 'A diet which is adequate for a man with a caloric requirement of 3,000 calories per day, simply cannot be assumed to cover the desirable nutritional supply for a low-caloric consumer.'

Sedentary schoolgirls, women office workers, elderly women, and, indeed, women generally, are liable to be short of vitamins and minerals, including calcium (Ca) and iron (Fe), says Dr Wretlind.

food bulging with vitamins and minerals, for shiny coats, wet noses and life-long bounce. Why feed your dog with Fit food, and then feed yourself and your family with rubbish?

Food poor in nourishment and heavy in calories means that in time you become ill, or fat, or ill *and* fat. This, of course, is where the 'health care' industry comes in●

**Note:** FAT TO FIT is not recommending Fit snacks on top of your 2,000 calories of Fit meals every day. If you eat a 250 calorie Fit snack, eat a smaller lunch or supper. Feel free to eat a hearty snack instead of a meal. But don't go hungry.

# THE POLITICS OF FOOD*

In October 1985, 'World in Action' broadcast 'The Great Food Scandal'. ITV's showcase current affairs programme showed that the truth about the harm Fat foods do to the national health has been hushed up by powerful people in Whitehall and the food manufacturing industry, working together in secret. The same week, Thames TV broadcast 'Good Enough To Eat?', about the contamination of our food by chemical additives. These programmes got twice the normal audience. Thames invited viewers to write in for a booklet on additives, and stopped reprinting after 35,000 requests had been received.

'Everybody knows that the wrong kind of food rots your teeth, and makes you overweight and constipated.' That's from the introduction to *You Are What You Eat*, the booklet accompanying the BBC TV series, which was part of a six-month BBC 'Food and Health Campaign'. On over-weight the booklet said 'don't bother about calorie counting ... If you're overweight eat plenty of vegetables, fruit and wholegrain food.' By the end of the six-part series on BBC1, 250 000 people had written in for the booklet.

In 1984, the Labour Party pledged itself to a good food policy. In November 1985, the Liberals went further and said that the Minister of Agriculture had 'a duty to encourage the production of food which is healthy'. So food and health is now even on the national political agenda.

What's going on? Why has food and health suddenly become a subject of intense public debate? And what's the matter with our food, anyway?

Two million people work for the food industry in Britain, if you count people in farming, distribution and catering. Any industry has a share of rogues, but the food industry as a whole has no interest in poisoning the population. Of course not. That's not the problem.

*For more on this topic read *The Food Scandal* (see booklist).

# ELEMENTAL BALANCE

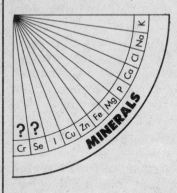

What are little girls, little boys and grown-up men and women made of? To a chemist, we consist almost entirely of just four of the elements or minerals found in nature. These are oxygen, carbon, hydrogen and nitrogen. Chemically, we are indeed what we eat – and drink – for ninety-six per cent of our bodies is made up of compounds of these four elements.

The other four per cent of us, chemically, is made up of many of the other elements found in nature, at least twelve of which are every bit as important for good health as are proteins, starches, fibres and essential fats. These are shown on the Wheel of Health.

We need nearly a gram both of calcium (Ca) and phosphorus (P) a day. These minerals work together with magnesium (Mg), to maintain strong, healthy bones and muscles.

With minerals the key word is balance. Minerals work together 'in partnership' in the body. And over a long period, imbalance is unhealthy. Various minerals can be 'competitive' or 'antagonistic', and thus eventually have a toxic effect. The notion, encouraged by people who sell pills, that you can't have too much of a good thing – the 'more the merrier', as it were – is simply untrue. All minerals can be toxic in excess.

This is not just an academic point. Potassium (K), sodium (Na) and chloride (Cl) are all essential nutrients, but ever since salt was extensively used as a preservative, people have consumed far too much sodium

The trouble started for us in Britain with the destruction of the peasantry. In a couple of generations, factory workers, crammed into slums and fed on the first, crude, mass-produced food, lost touch with the earth and its fruits. In the nineteenth century the national food supply became loaded with hard fats and processed sugars, white bread, jams and confectionery. These were – and are – all 'good' commodities, from the manufacturer's point of view. 'Good'

and chloride (which is what salt is made of). Average intake of sodium nowadays is ten or twenty times more than the body needs. Worse still, the British food supply is short of potassium, found in abundance in fresh foods, but lost in processing. The resulting gross imbalance between sodium and potassium is likely to be a major cause of high blood pressure and strokes.

The other six minerals on the Wheel are known as 'trace elements', which merely means they are required in tiny amounts. Iron (Fe), zinc (Zn) and copper (Cu) should also work in harmony with each other. We've all heard that iron (and calcium) are vital to health, because they were officially 'scheduled' nearly half a century ago. But anaemia (lack of iron) and weak bones (lack of calcium) still remain public health problems in Britain.

Of the 'unscheduled' minerals, still not officially recognised in Britain as significant, zinc is one of the most important, especially to women.

Severe lack of zinc is known to cause what in infants is called 'failure to thrive': it's vital for growth. So females who are very short of zinc may suffer slow growth in adolescence, loss of appetite, lost periods, no sex drive, depression, stretch marks, slow-healing flesh, vulnerability to infection and – a special mark of zinc deficiency – a literal loss of taste for food.

Any woman who is short of zinc and takes iron pills, for anaemia or in pregnancy, will suffer more, since, like other minerals, iron in excess is an 'antagonist': it will drive zinc out of the body.

The three remaining minerals on the wheel are iodine (I) which protects against goitre; selenium (Se) which probably protects against cancers; and chromium (Cr) which probably protects against diabetes. Figures for selenium and chromium content of foods are not comprehensive, hence the queries (?) on the Wheels.

**Note:** for an explanation of the standards used in compiling the Wheels, see pages 181–86.

commodities keep for a long time: they don't go bad.

But really good food does go bad. This is because it has life in it. From the health point of view any foodstuff that does not readily decay in a short period of time, is suspect. And this is why there is a conflict of interest between the manufacturer and the consumer. If people prefer Fit food and are prepared to demand it, then the clash between industry and the citizen is minimized. But in Britain we have

# ANOREXIA

Here is a new horror word. A young woman who is diagnosed as 'anorexic' is seen not exactly as mad, but certainly as having 'mental problems'. Lots of books have been written about anorexia or 'eating disorders'. Most studies see them as neuroses through which young women refuse to become adult or, alternatively, reject the rules of society.

Unfortunately few doctors of medicine have any knowledge of nutrition, which is not part of the 'modern' medical syllabus. However, a number of scientists and doctors who have studied nutrition now believe that anorexia is not a mental condition, but a disease caused by gross deficiency of good food.

The argument goes as follows. The body needs nourishment, not just energy from food. Anybody who eats a typical amount of highly processed food, including snacks and junk drinks, and who also under-eats, is liable to be very under-nourished. If the individual also decides to go on calorie-cutting diets, her body is liable to become severely short of nourishment. The key nutrient looks like being the trace element zinc (Zn – see page 90) which is crucial to growth.

Zinc is stored in muscle. (Meat, being muscle, is a good source of zinc.) A body desperate for zinc may in effect feed upon itself – hence compulsive starvation to release zinc from the body. This also explains why anorexics often over-exercise, which is another way the body breaks down muscle tissue.

Anybody who is severely anorexic is short of every kind of nourishment and needs urgent medical help. But in the early stages, anorexics should try kicking out all junk products and eating only highly nutritious food.

been trained to accept cheap and convenient food: and this means Fat food, a more sophisticated version of the stuff that people suffered from in Victorian days, and in the 1930s. Indeed, analysed on the Wheel of Health, food as supplied to the working class in the 1930s was in some vital respects not as bad as food in supermarkets today.

Ironically, cheap food is bad policy for all but the biggest producers in the industry. Britain's food manufacture is dominated by a small number of gigantic conglomerate firms, highly capitalized, and very profitable. But the British food industry as a whole is not in such good shape. Tens of thousands of small firms have gone to the wall. Bakers, greengrocers, fishmongers and butchers have vanished from the high streets. Small farmers have gone bankrupt and agribusiness employs fewer and fewer people on the land. Every year a static population spends less and less on food because the customer doesn't value cheapened food much, at any price. Highly processed Fat food is rotten value for money.

Be that as it may, the manufacturers of highly processed food in Britain are well organized. The Food and Drink Federation (FDF) is the trade organization set up to protect the interests of the manufacturer of highly processed food in Westminster, Whitehall and Brussels. It is highly effective. The FDF is allied with other trade organizations, such as the Bacon and Meat Manufacturers (BMMA), the Cake and Biscuit ·Alliance (CBA), the Cocoa, Chocolate and Confectionery Alliance (CCCA), and the Snack, Nut and Crisp Manufacturers' Association (SNACMA).

Outside the FDF there are the Sugar Bureau, the Butter Information Council, and the Salt Data Centre, who circulate journalists, doctors and other opinion-formers with documents, some under the heading 'Diet and Health', putting in the good word for sugar, butter and salt.

Do the manufacturers of highly processed food get their way? In May 1985, a debate on the confectionery industry was concluded by MAFF Minister, Peggy Fenner. 'I conclude by congratulating the confectionery industry,' she said, 'and I assure it and the House of our concern to ensure a propitious climate for its continued success.' In 1985 £312,000,000 tax was paid to the Government by the confectionery trade.

Your journey from Fat to Fit can start as from your next brisk walk to the shops, but if you want Britain to have a good food supply you will have to fight for it.

The move to Fit, healthy food has to involve moves towards

a healthy food industry. But, as with any national change for the better, an industry reconstructed with the national health in mind would mean a new Government committed to our good health.

Now's the time to convince politicians that commitment to a healthy national food supply is a vote-winner. You can make a start by writing to your local MP. And next time, put your vote where your mouth is●

# THE ECONOMICS OF DIETING

People who want their friendly neighbourhood doctor to solve their overweight problem are now being encouraged to ask 'got any gum, chum?'. Guar is In. It's a gum from the seeds of the cluster bean plant (cyamopsis tetragonolobus) which is classified as a type of soluble fibre. In December 1985 there was even a conference at the Royal Society of Medicine entitled 'Guar: Where Do We Go From Here?'

Medics are keen on guar. It seems to be a good treatment for high levels of fats in the blood, blood-sugar variation, high blood pressure, and adult-onset diabetes. Word has got around that there's gold in them thar beans.

What nobody at the Royal Society of Medicine conference got round to mentioning, however, is that there are rather more familiar and accessible forms of soluble fibre. Oats, for a start. If guar is good for high blood pressure, diabetes, and excess fat, etc., so is porridge. But from the business point of view, porridge is a dead loss. It's cheap.

Fat farms are one of the most successful bits of business ever devised. Country houses scattered over the Home Counties charge hotel rates for what can indeed be comfortable and relaxing accommodation: the difference being that you don't get fed. You get a bill, but if you ask for a meal the answer's a lemon. Some 'health farms' *are* now worthy of the name, and offer Fit food and activity.

Others charge more for eating less, and every year the fatties return, like old lags. In time no doubt they'll be offered a short sharp dose of cyamopsis tetragonolobus.

Down-market, for those who can only dream of fat farms, there are magazines with advertisements for varieties of 'slimming' processed foods with added air or water. 'Slimming' products are subtly presented as part-food, part-medicine. Some are indeed made with chemicals. Others are Fit foods at a Fat price, or else made to look faintly cranky●

# THE DIETING REGIMES

In my dieting days there was plenty of choice on the diet front. There was the Scarsdale Diet (high protein), the Stillman Diet (high protein again), the Beverly Hills Medical Diet (high carbohydrate), the 'This Slimming Business' diet (low carbohydrate), and the 'Eat Fat and Grow Slim' diet (high fat). Later there was the Beverly Hills Diet (exotic) and the F-Plan Diet (high fibre). Whatever the content of these diet régimes, in principle they all amount to the same thing: calorie-cutting.

Now, cutting calories has gone high-tech, with 'micro-diets', also known as 'very low calorie diets' or VLCDs for short. These cut the calories down to around 300 a day, and supply protein, vitamins and minerals in powder form. Micro-diets are marketed with zeal by satisfied customers who are called 'counsellors'. You may have tried a micro-diet, or an old-fashioned calorie-cutting diet. But does calorie-cutting work for you? Check out your own experience by filling in the questionnaire on the next page.

With food, think quality not quantity. Think quantity with activity. The only diet plan that can possibly work for you, life-long, is a plan you make part of your life and enjoy life-long●

# DIETS YOU HAVE KNOWN

As a slimmer, is this the first book you've picked up? Or are you a seasoned campaigner with a boxful of old dieting books and magazines? If so, here is your big chance to reminisce.

Think back. Remember when you tried the Scarsdale diet, or the F-Plan. Locate the year when you were a Weight Watcher, or followed the Yudkin 'Slimming Business', or went to a fat farm or on a fast. If you've tried a micro-diet, note that down too.

If you can remember, note down your weight before and after the diet. Never mind if you can't remember exactly; guess if necessary. Then look down all the 'before' weights in the left hand column, and all the 'after' weights in the right hand column. I've also left room for you to enter your weight and waist measurement before and after your calorie-cutting days. That done, decide for yourself: is now the time you decide to go from Fat to Fit, forever?

| | Year | Weight | | Waist | |
|---|---|---|---|---|---|
| | | Before | After | Before | After |
| BCC* | | | | | |
| Atkins | | | | | |
| Beverly Hills | | | | | |
| Cambridge | | | | | |
| F-Plan | | | | | |
| Fasting | | | | | |
| Fat farm | | | | | |
| Herbalife | | | | | |
| Scarsdale | | | | | |
| Stillman | | | | | |
| Univite | | | | | |
| Weight Watchers | | | | | |
| Yudkin | | | | | |
| Other (name) | | | | | |
| Other (name) | | | | | |
| ACC** | | | | | |
| Does cutting calories work for you? | Yes | | | No | |
| * Before Calorie Cutting (your pre-dieting days)    ** After Calorie Cutting | | | | | |

# FAT TO FIT

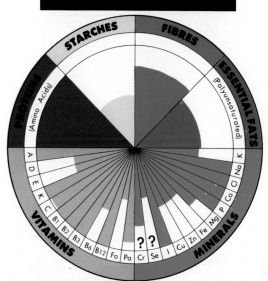

# YOUR AT-A-GLANCE GUIDE

**L**ook around in the shops at the labels of packaged foods. **Four fifths of the British food supply is processed, crammed with machine-made, 'refined', fats, sugars and starches** ● The Wheel of Health above shows what is missing from the British food supply. If you eat the average sort of everyday food, this Wheel applies to you. The Wheel for a fully nourishing and satisfying diet would have every one of its segments completely filled in. On the following pages Fat and Fit versions of three typical, everyday meals are compared

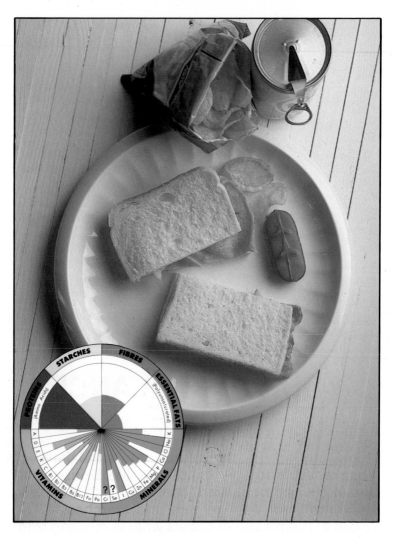

Here are two sandwich bar lunches. You can immediately see from the Wheels for each lunch that a couple of wholemeal sandwiches, plus yoghurt and whole fruits, is the healthy choice. Saturated fats (from the bacon, margarine or butter, and crisps) with other fats and sugars (from confectionery) have driven goodness out of the lunch shown in this photograph ●

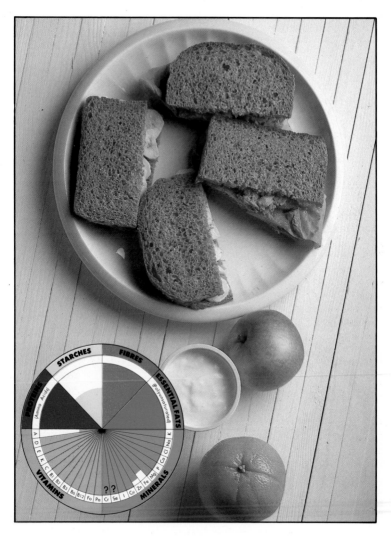

This is the filling and satisfying lunch. It is literally twice the size of the bacon sandwich'n'no-cal drink choice, so it will fill you up and stop mid-afternoon cravings. It is also a lot tastier. But it contains exactly the same 700 calories – about one third of the energy a woman uses in a day. As you can see from its Wheel, it is an almost perfect balanced meal. Turn to page 21 for the full story of a good lunch ●

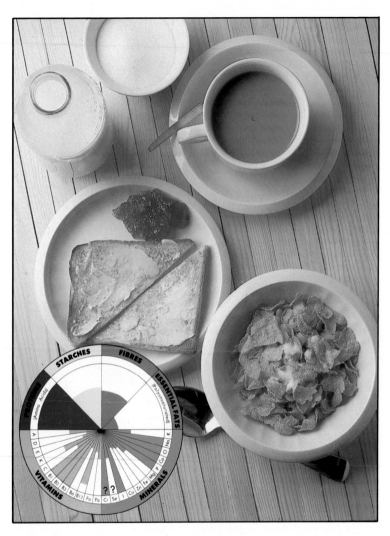

What's the first thing you do in the morning if you want to lose fat? Skip breakfast, right? Wrong! The first step on the way to a new, slim you is to enjoy a nourishing and filling breakfast. The choice on this page isn't all bad: after all, manufacturers add back some vitamins and minerals to processed cereals and bread. But look at the Wheel and see what has been lost ●

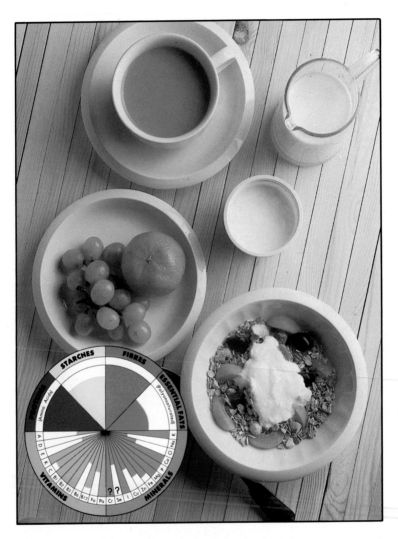

The great thing about muesli, when it's sugar-free and made from whole grains, is that it's crammed with goodness and made delicious and even more nourishing by adding low-fat yoghurt, a little dried fruit and masses of fresh fruit. This Fit breakfast contains the same 400 calories as the fatty and sugary processed choice, yet it's nutrient-rich. For more Fit breakfasts, turn to page 33 ●

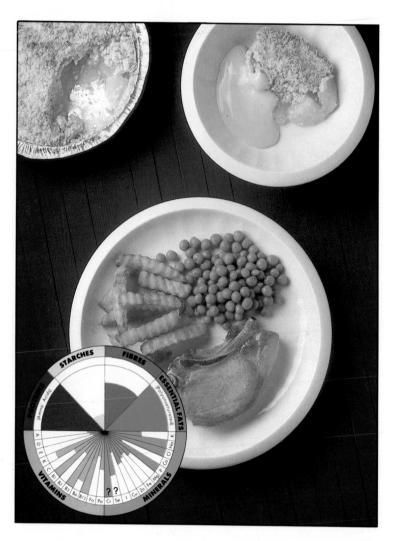

The Wheels of Health on these two pages show a spectacular contrast in quality between two evening meals, both easy to prepare, both adaptable to one or two people or to a family and both including meat and vegetables with fruit to follow. This chop, chips, peas and apple crumble meal has some quality, but its fats and sugars are liable to make you fat and leave you hungry ●

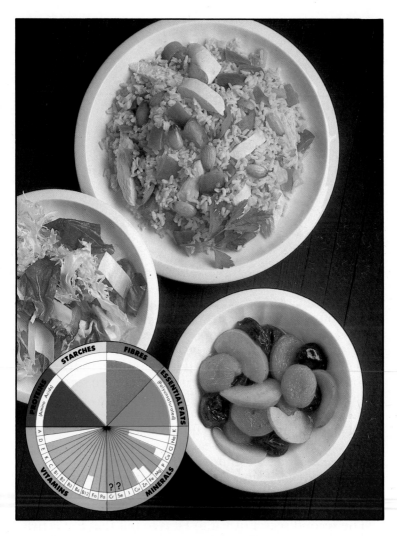

Look at the size of this supper! This great plateful of risotto should stick to your ribs, leaving you full and satisfied, but it contains exactly the same calories – 900 – as the chop'n'chips meal. This meal is twice as heavy, but the weight is in natural fibres and water, which won't make you fat. Wholegrain cereals and whole vegetables, salads and fruit, make Fit meals. Now turn to page 49 ●

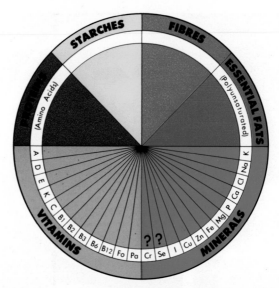

The only reliable and permanent way from Fat to Fit is to enjoy your fill of whole, fresh food. Forget about cutting calories – look forward to the pleasures of delicious, nourishing food, maybe for the first time in your adult life.

People who try to lose extra fat are trained to fear food; to think of it as some kind of enemy. Here are some of the misleading ideas put into the minds of dieters:

- I musn't be greedy. Feeling full is bad.
- Feeling empty is good. Hunger is a virtue.
- I must avoid food and eat only when hungry.
- When I don't feel hungry, I must not eat.

The way from Fat to Fit is twofold. First, transform the quality of the food you eat. Kick out every kind of highly processed food. Instead, eat your fill of whole, fresh food.

The second secret of Fat to Fit is to put that lost activity back into your life. Around the turn of the century, before the age of the car, people used around 300–500 more calories each day through their everyday activity. You could do the same.

The full account of how to restore your lost energy begins on page 175. The Wheel of Health on this page is your goal; it shows what fully Fit good food looks like ●

# FAT TO FIT

## 6

# WELCOME TO THE WEEKEND

**W**hat would you rather do at the weekend? Lie around feeling miserable? Or have a big lunch, maybe with friends, and then take a walk in the park or the countryside? ● Now's the time for plenty of good food, and plenty of fresh air: invite friends round and delight them with an old-fashioned, Great British cooked breakfast ● More good news, about the wholefood fats that make you fit ● Eating and activity in pregnancy; getting Fit for two ● And have fun being energetic outdoors, at all seasons of the year

Healthy food. What do these words mean to you? What words and images swim into your mind when you think of 'healthy food'? Close your eyes, relax, and think . . .

Cranks. Nut rissoles. Muesli eaten out of a wok. Foreign muck. 'Food Lentilists'. Royal jelly. Decaffeinated coffee. Open-toed sandals. Garlic perles. 'Real men don't eat quiche'. Muddy vegetables. Soya milk. Anaemic women in shops selling ginseng, kelp tablets, 'vitamin B17' and mudbath packs. Bran. Tea that smells funny. Rabbit food. Adukiburgers. Bean sprouts.

Is this something like your idea of healthy food? It used

to be mine. I was wrong. Dead wrong. In particular, I used to assume that eating healthy food would be a bit of a chore. It was imprinted on my mind that real food, delicious food, food to feast from, was unhealthy ('naughty but nice' as the advertisements say). I resisted paying attention to food and health because I didn't want to start eating dull, heavy, tasteless food. Who would? If the choice is good health or good fun, lots of people will choose fun.

Here are three of the myths which have been stated again and again in calorie-cutting diet books. I've mentioned them elsewhere in FAT TO FIT, but they bear repeating:

● **Myth: most people in Britain eat too much.**
  Truth: most people in Western countries, including Britain, do not eat enough. Typically, people become fat not because of greed, but because machines have made them sedentary. People who exercise regularly can eat as much good food as they like and not gain fat.

● **Myth: carbohydrates make you fat.**
  Truth: processed, 'refined' sugars added to food are Fat food. But by total contrast, whole starchy foods like wholegrain bread, are Fit food, full of nourishment. Sugars in natural form are also Fit food. Whole food is good for you. It is highly processed carbohydrates that make you fat.

● **Myth: fat is bad for health.**
  Truth: almost everybody in Western countries eats far too much fat, and, in particular, saturated fats, from highly processed foods, and from meat and dairy products. Saturated fats are indeed Fat food. But essential fats, from fish, game, cereals, nuts and seeds, *are* vital to health.

Now, if you consider these three truths not separately, but together, they show that the calorie-cutting diet books have got it all wrong. Indeed, they show that conventional

# THE CHOICE IS YOURS

**BRUNCH**

| | FAT 700 calories | FIT (1) 700 calories | FIT (2) 700 calories |
|---|---|---|---|
| | Egg (1, fried) Bacon (1 rasher, grilled) Sausage (1, fried) Tomatoes (3½oz, fried) | Kidneys (7oz, fried) Mushrooms (3½oz, fried) Tomatoes (3½oz, fried in 1 tbsp corn oil) Sweetcorn (3½oz) | Salmon (2oz tinned) French beans (3½oz), Butter beans (3½oz), Tomatoes (3½oz), Olives (1oz) Chicory (1oz), Orange (2oz), Watercress (1oz), Celery (1oz) French dressing (2tbsps) Carrots (3½oz, raw), White cabbage (3½oz) |
| | Bread (1 slice white, fried) | Potatoes (sauté, 7oz) | Bread (2 slices, wholemeal) |
| | Coffee (1 cup), sugar (1 tsp), milk (full fat) | Orange juice (1 glass) | Wine (1 glass, white) |
| Saturated fats Sugars Salt Additives | HEAVY LIGHT HEAVY HEAVY | LIGHT LIGHT LIGHT* LIGHT | LIGHT LIGHT LIGHT* LIGHT |
| Proteins Starches Fibres Essential fats | SUPER-RICH POOR POOR POOR/MEDIUM | SUPER-RICH POOR/MEDIUM RICH RICH | SUPER-RICH POOR SUPER-RICH RICH |
| Vitamin D Vitamin E | POOR POOR | POOR MEDIUM | SUPER-RICH RICH |
| Calcium (Ca) Magnesium (Mg) | POOR POOR | POOR RICH | RICH RICH |

* if not added

Key to terms used here and on Wheels of Health: page 199.
Fit brunch recipes: Chapter 9.

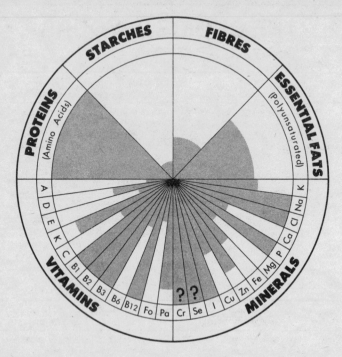

● **Fat brunch: egg, bacon, sausage, tomato, fried bread.** There is plenty of nourishment in bacon and eggs, and in tomatoes too. True, bacon is very salty, but if you kicked the sausage and fried bread out of this brunch, used good oil, and had a couple of eggs and a lot more tomatoes and bread, its 700 calories would be fit for an occasional treat. But this fry-up is soaked in fats and won't fill you. (Menu: page 107.)

wisdom, as reflected in textbooks and officially approved statements about food and health in the last half-century, up until a few years ago, has been wrong too.

The rationale of most diet books is 'high-protein, low-calorie'. The one great thing about the 'F-Plan' is that Audrey Eyton made starches and fibres popular, and moved slimmers away from steak-and-lettuce-leaf régimes. But the 'F-Plan' still relies on calorie-cutting, just

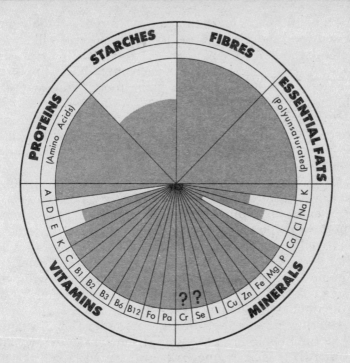

● **Fit brunch: kidneys, mushrooms, tomatoes, sauté potatoes.** Surprise, surprise, eh? A big fried breakfast that is Fit! Bet you've never seen *that* in a dieting book! The fact is that a genuine, traditional, Great British breakfast of kidneys, mushrooms and potatoes is super-rich in many vitamins and minerals. Amaze your friends by inviting them around for this 700 calorie feast. (Menu: page 107. Recipe: page 168.)

like the Stillman and Scarsdale diets. One popular diet book that takes proper account of the value of activity is the Pritikin plan, much better known in America than in Britain. But the key for everybody (including slimmers) to remember, is that the healthiest food is whole, fresh food, and plenty of it. The worst food for health is highly processed food; the more highly processed, the Fatter it will be.

These messages make the manufacturers of highly processed food sad. But there it is. Food scientists will always defend food processing, because their job is to process food. And to date, people in government have supported the food scientists and the giant food manufacturers, although times are changing now.

If the problem is highly processed food, did our grandparents and great-grandparents eat better food than most people now? If they could get hold of fresh food, and if they had enough to eat, the answer is yes.

My father comes from Poplar. In his young day, families sat down in the afternoon to the Cockney Tea. This was a big meal: with lashings of tea and mounds of coarse bread (there were plenty of local master bakers in those days) there'd be great platters of fruits from the sea. What choice! Cockles, mussels, whelks and eels from the Thames estuary; crabs and sometimes oysters from the Essex coast; bloaters, kippers, and herring in other forms, from the East Anglian ports.

Herring, now wrongly despised, is super-rich in vitamin D, all the B vitamins, potassium (K), magnesium (Mg) and iron (Fe). It is also super-rich in essential fats. Take my word for it: herring is very Fit food. So are expensive deep-sea and river fish, like salmon and trout, and cheap fish like sardines, sprats and anchovies. My local fishmonger sells sprats for forty-five pence a pound.

The equivalent of the cooked Tea today is what Americans call Brunch – breakfast and lunch rolled into one, ideal for weekends. Feast on fish for brunch as in our salmon and salad meal (page 170), or enjoy another traditional British meal: kidneys and mushrooms, with tomatoes, featured in the Wheel on page 111. If you like bacon with kidneys, that's fine too, but be choosy when you buy bacon. Insist on a lean cut, use it sparingly and grill it.

High-quality wholegrain bread, cut thick, is one Fit accompaniment to a Great British brunch. So, I am very happy to tell you, are sauté potatoes. If you cut potatoes

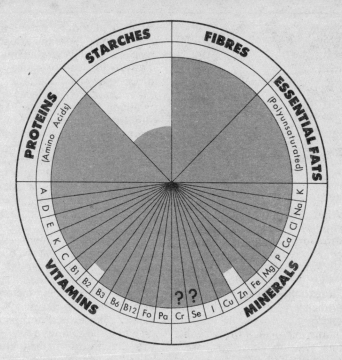

● **Fit brunch: salmon and salads.** Apart from starch, this is an almost perfectly balanced meal. Salmon is super-rich in essential fats, vitamin D and minerals, carrots bulge with vitamin A (carotene), oranges supply vitamin C, and the bread and salads fill other corners. Notice the generous helping of oil in the French dressing, and the wine. For a very special treat have fresh rather than tinned salmon. (Menu: page 107. Recipe: page 170.)

thick, par-boil them first, and fry them in very hot, good quality oil, high in polyunsaturates, you will set yourself up for a long, brisk walk in the afternoon. A word about cooking-oil. Never use blended oil. Corn, safflower, sunflower, soya and sesame are good choices. So is high-quality olive oil.

The upper-class, Great British breakfast was also a Fit feast, once upon a time. What went wrong in Victorian

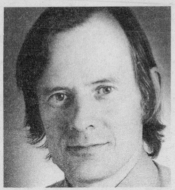

What's wrong with our food supply? **Professor Michael Crawford** (above), of the Biochemistry Department at the Nuffield Institute, Regent's Park, is in no doubt. 'The industrialized West has created artificially protein-rich and energy-rich foods' he told me 'at the expense of the essential fats. We now know that essential fats are directly involved in the development, maintenance and health of the nervous and vascular systems of the body.'

In early 1985, Dr Crawford organized a world conference on essential fats, in London. A highlight was a feast of fish, as eaten in London down the ages, from Roman soused mussels, to a Georgian mackerel in gooseberry sauce, to the Cockney Tea (page 110).

Dr Crawford believes in traditional food. He has worked with tribal peoples in Africa, and points out that free-living animals are lean; and more important, their bodies are rich in essential fats. Fish from the deep sea are now just about the only 'wild' food we eat, and are super-rich in essential fats, vitamins and minerals.

By contrast, the intensively-reared animals we eat are bred to be obese, and their fat is solid – heavily saturated. 'The present concept in factory-farming is like keeping a healthy man in bed and feeding him 5,000 calories a day.'

Dr Crawford is fiercely critical of government-approved policy of feeding babies with lots of full-fat cows' milk. He believes this effects not just the body, but the brain. So we could be breeding a new race of beefy, stupid people, liable to die young.

and Edwardian days was that food was cooked according to recipes from corrupted editions of Mrs Beeton's *Household Management*, compiled and published long after her death. These recipes were packed with fats and sugars, and the urban middle classes started to eat great quantities of Fat food – their equivalent of the business lunches and dinner parties that make the modern middle class bunged up, fat, and diseased in middle age.

By utter contrast, wealthy, landed people and their guests in Edwardian days could and did eat fabulously Fit food, particularly game, fish and fruit and vegetables grown on the estate. And you can eat food fit for a king without being a lord, nowadays. Two of my local butchers stock rabbit and hare, pigeon and pheasant, wild duck and grouse. If you like eating flesh, all you need to know for health is that the animal itself was Fit and active in its life. The flesh of all animals intensively reared on grassland is highly saturated with fat: all such animals are unfit and unhealthy, as you will be if you sit and stand around all day. By contrast the hunter and the hunted animal are, or should be, fit and lean.

Next time you think of healthy food, don't think of nut rissoles and bran. Think of a Great British breakfast, and eat it for brunch●

# PEOPLE WHO DESERVE THE BEST

Here is an Irish joke. An Irish student of nutrition was once asked 'is there malnutrition in Ireland?' The answer he gave was 'there is no malnutrition in Ireland, except among pregnant and lactating women, babies, growing children, adolescents, the elderly, tinkers, drunks, and poor people.'

This 'joke' points to what is officially known as 'the nutritional status of "at-risk groups"'. 'Malnutrition', of course, does not mean starvation, but, literally, bad nutrition. 'At-risk groups' are those groups of people in any population who are most likely to suffer from bad food. The official line is that the food supply is fine (and getting better), public health is fine (and getting better) and that there need be no concern about food as a cause of ill-health, except among 'at-risk groups'.

In Britain, the official line has been demolished by Professor John Catford in a *British Medical Journal* review. Dr

# FATS:
# THE FACTS

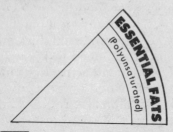

ESSENTIAL FATS
(polyunsaturated)

**T**hree messages about fats have now been put across in a big way. First, there is far too much fat in the food supply. Second, fats make you fat. Third, saturated fats cause heart attacks.

These messages are essentially true. Certainly, as with sugars, the less saturated fats you eat, the better. Around one fifth of the calories in the British food supply now, is in the form of saturated fats, and another one fifth in the form of processed, added sugars. This means that forty per cent of the food in the shops is empty, or trash calories.

Saturated fats (also called 'saturated fatty acids' or SFAs) are hard at normal temperatures. Fat from domesticated animals is highly saturated. So is coconut and palm oil.

Why, then, didn't the people who enjoyed the roast beef of Olde England, keel over from heart attacks? First, because the fat of animals left to roam free is less saturated than that of animals that are penned up. Second, because for all but the rich, meat was for special, feast days. Third, the fact is that the nobility, who gorged on meats and sweetmeats, *did* get fat (as you can see from portraits), and *did* keel over from strokes and heart attacks.

In any case, good fresh meat isn't a health hazard unless you actually gorge on it. The problem, as ever, is highly processed food, including meat products like the infamous Great British sausage, crammed with extra cheap, saturated fats. In processing, fats are made highly saturated by a process called 'hydrogenation'. This isn't because

Catford has shown that rates of premature death from a number of major diseases, of which a food supply high in fats, sugars and salt is a major cause, are now higher in Britain than in any other European country. In the case of heart disease the rate is higher than anywhere else in the world. The commonest disease caused by Fat food, after tooth decay and constipation is, of course, overweight, or more correctly, 'overfat'. It's agreed that one in every

WELCOME TO THE WEEKEND

the manufacturers want to turn you from a consumer into a patient, but simply because saturated fats are stable: they keep, they have a long shelf-life, they don't seep out all over the packet.

Fats are liable to make you fat simply because all types of fat and oil are intensely concentrated forms of energy (calories). People in Britain and America consume around four ounces (over 100 grams) of fats a day, of which half are saturated. In processed form, fats drive nourishment out.

So that's the bad news about fats. The good news, for everybody who wants to get Fit is that other types of fat are positively good for you.

The civilizations of Greece and southern Italy were created by people whose cuisine was and still is, based on olive oil, which is uniquely high in monounsaturated fats. And all **un**saturated fat is benign.

Fats from whole foods such as grain, nuts and seeds, and from fit animals such as game and fish, are all rich in poly-unsaturated fatty acids (PUFAs for short). Certain PUFAs are known as essential fats (or EFAs, short for essential fatty acids). They have also been called vitamin F, because they are vital to health and life. This is why they are included on the Wheel of Health.

Dr Hugh Sinclair and Professor Michael Crawford, two world authorities on fats, point out that the soft tissue of the brain and central nervous system is mostly made of essential fats. It may be that the energy and enterprise of hunters and fishermen is nourished from birth by game and fish, rich in essential fats. By contrast, a nation whose babies are fed on full-fat cows' milk is breeding big bodies but, perhaps, small minds.

The British food supply is poor in essential fats. To fill the Wheel, essential fats should supply six and a half per cent of all calories. This is easily achieved if you use nothing but good quality, unblended, high-polyunsaturated oils.

three adults in Britain is overfat, and that after the age of forty the figure is around one in every two, with around one in ten people frankly obese – so fat that the quality of their lives is spoiled, and their life-expectation shortened.

The people suffering most from Fat food are those groups identified in the Irish joke, and also the unemployed, and people in Scotland, Wales, the north of England and Northern Ireland. Additionally, there is now

# ALCOHOL

**W**hat about booze? Alcohol hasn't figured much in these pages, apart from the occasional reference to pubs, or a glass of wine being a pleasant addition to a Fit meal. Is there anything to be said for it?

The simple answer is: think of alcohol the same way you think of processed sugars. Both are empty calories. Both are potentially addictive. Both are a direct cause of disease. For many people, childhood sweets become adult drinks.

Just as with processed sugars, an occasional drink, as well as being agreeable, is not going to shorten your life. As with other foods, the important thing is to insist on high quality. Enjoy a glass of real ale, or honest wine, from time to time, but refuse the refuse.

Heavy drinking is almost as destructive as heavy smoking. For health, it's best not to drink at all. One or two drinks (amounting to a pint of beer, or a large glass of wine, or a double measure of spirits) every other day or so, won't damage you. But if you need to drink every day, you should be concerned, as you should be if you need confectionery or cola drinks every day.

The confectionery and alcohol manufacturers like to sponsor sports events, to give the impression that really Fit people *need* sweets or booze. This is a load of rubbish. The energy that Fit people need comes best from nourishing food. Whenever you notice a food or drink manufacturer boasting about the energy content of their product, they're promoting empty calories.

The time for women to say 'no' to alcohol is when they are thinking of having a child. For a woman, the best possible opportunity to eat and drink nothing but Fit food, is while preparing to eat and drink for two. This is also the time for Mere Males to express their sympathy by laying off the booze too.

good evidence that babies, children and adolescents of all classes, everywhere in Britain, are liable to suffer from clusters of disorders and diseases caused by Fat food.

People in government are aware that Fat food is a major public health problem. From time to time, government departments commission surveys of 'at-risk groups'. In recent years these have included surveys of the nutritional status of eleven to fourteen-year-olds, fifteen to twenty-five-year-olds, pregnant women, and the elderly. These reports have been delayed, redrafted, got 'stuck in the computer', been eventually published in obscure journals, or have been just suppressed.

You're probably reading this book because you want to get rid of your own excess fat. I want to encourage you to see that excess fat is just one result of Fat food. If you are a mother of growing children, or thinking of becoming a mother; if you are adolescent, or, alternatively, if you are really short of money; if you live alone or are elderly, then your own health is only one reason for you to value whole food and fresh air.

Above all, the time to care about becoming Fit is when you decide to have a baby. If your family doctor understands about Fit food, you are in luck. If not, seek out your local community dietitian: find her (it's usually a her) by looking up your local health authority in the Yellow Pages. Take FAT TO FIT with you: if your doctor or dietitian says that a 'normal, balanced, varied diet' is all you need, without defining what they mean, find another doctor or dietitian●

# MADE FOR WALKING

What happens to domestic, farm or zoo animals that are kept penned up? They become fat, constipated, listless and ill. By contrast, a dog that is walked – or run – and is fed good food, stays sleek and vigorous, and has the best chance of dying in good health of old age. The same is true of people.

Professor Per-Olof Åstrand, from Sweden, probably knows more about the value of activity in everyday life than anybody else alive today. In 1983, he gave a keynote address to a conference, 'Exercise, Health, Medicine', held in Britain at Lilleshall Hall, a centre owned by the Sports Council. 'We are directly descended from people who rested when well-fed,' he said, 'but whose healthy existence depended on a large amount of vigorous exercise.' For tens of thousands of years our ancestors walked for hours each day, to find food, using bodies made for walking.

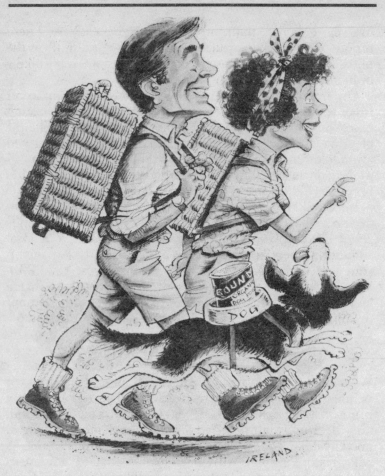

After all, said Dr Åstrand 'we all know that a dog needs exercise, so if the dog needs exercise, surely we do too? So, we should all take the dog for a walk – even if we don't have one!'

And therein lies the problem for most adults in our society – lack of activity, and above all, walking. In my father's young day, outdoor recreation was universally popular. Young couples and families living in London took the underground train to the end of the line, and went on picnic-rambles with rucksacks at weekends. This was the hey-day of the Youth Hostel, used as a base by holiday hikers in Britain and throughout Europe.

Of course, not everybody spent their two summer weeks off work walking up alps. But these were the pre-central heating days. Sitting at home wasn't always comfortable, so people generated their own heat, which is what the body is designed to do. And these were the days of the train and bus, which everybody used, to go to work, or to the shops, but which do not provide door-to-door service. It was normal to walk a mile to the train station and then another mile to work. And there were no suburban supermarkets with car parks and trolley service: you walked to the shops and carried your own bags.

Times have changed. I recall going to Newcastle one sunny, summer day, to take part in a programme on Metro Radio, which is located just outside the city. I started to walk in the general direction of the radio station, and every ten minutes or so, stopped people and asked them how far I had to go. Only one person, an elderly man, said 'it's forty minutes walk away'. Everybody else had no idea. They said 'have you got a car?' or 'ooh, it's too far to walk', or simply didn't know.

This isn't a story against the people of Newcastle. Try it for yourself. Get a map of the area where you live. Mark a spot three miles away from where you live, then walk towards it, and ask people how far away it is. You'll get some funny answers. People have stopped walking. Another example. A colleague of mine, who regards me as a bit of an expert, telephoned me and explained that he was over forty and was beginning to feel the need for some regular exercise. 'Walk across the parks to work' I said. It's a journey of three and a half miles across the parks, after which he could jump on a bus. 'I couldn't do that', he said, 'I haven't got the time'. 'Well' I said, 'you could walk and think at the same time.' My basic advice to every able-bodied person is: walk briskly for an hour every day●

# STEPPING IT OUT

Below are listed ten outdoor activities and recreations that can be enjoyed in a leisurely way, or energetically. Plus there are a couple of rows for you to fill in any activity of yours not on the list. If you have babies, children or pets, there's room for them too. Don't just tick the boxes. Write 'Love', 'Like', 'OK', 'Dislike' or 'Hate' instead. For example, if you shop every day and don't mind it, write 'OK' in the left-hand column. First, though, rate your overall level of outdoor activity.

Compared with other people I know, I would say that during the week, at weekends and on holiday I am:

| Weekdays | Very active | Average | Inactive |
|---|---|---|---|
| Weekends | Very active | Average | Inactive |
| Holidays | Very active | Average | Inactive |

I would rate the level of my activity and recreation, and how I feel about it, as follows:

| | Daily | Every other day | Weekly | Monthly | Never |
|---|---|---|---|---|---|
| Decorating | | | | | |
| Gardening | | | | | |
| Shopping | | | | | |
| Walking | | | | | |
| Washing (car) | | | | | |
| Badminton | | | | | |
| Cycling | | | | | |
| Dancing | | | | | |
| Hiking | | | | | |
| Tennis | | | | | |
| Other (name) | | | | | |
| Other (name) | | | | | |
| Babies | | | | | |
| Children | | | | | |
| Dog | | | | | |

# FAT TO FIT

## 7

# TIME FOR A PARTY

**F**aced with a dinner party what do you do? Say 'no'? Or 'to hell with it' – and get fat and ill? Good news for sociable slimmers: if you choose Fit food, the bigger the feast, the better ● Cookbooks you can trust ● How to give children the best start at school and at home ● Why the obesity 'experts' are blind with science, and why 'sweet fat' with additives makes you fat and ill ● Plenty of good food, and plenty of fresh air: the foundation for enjoying a long and healthy life, and the way from Fit to Superfit

Think of all the festival days of your life. There are the red-letter days we all share in common: Christmas and Boxing Day above all, and New Year. There are all the birthdays in your life: your own, and those of your family and close friends. And there are the special high days: marriage, a promotion at work, the signing of a contract, a prize won, a welcome or farewell for friends. What all these occasions have in common is feasting, for, after all, 'festival' means 'feast day'. A feast is what we offer our nearest and dearest, to mark the special relationship. 'Dinner party' is the phrase nowadays.

Feasting is the modern slimmer's version of Sin. A Good

slimmer stays away from parties or, like a saint in a brothel, prods the temptation on offer, and says 'no'. A Bad slimmer says 'just this once', tucks in, and wakes up vowing 'never again', yet longing for more.

Half-starving yourself in an attempt to lose fat is an odd business, if you stop to think about it. As a mass social phenomenon, it's pretty much confined to the rich, white Protestant parts of the world. Is this because Catholics and others with a religion have deeper things about which to feel sinful and tempted, and bigger things to repent?

If you drew a map of those countries in the world whose women's magazines regularly carry cover stories on calorie-cutting, and another map marking those countries whose food supply features not-only saturated fats and processed sugars but also highly sophisticated combinations of 'sweet fat' with additives, the two maps would probably be identical. And it is only in those same Western and Westernized countries that people worry about feasting and, to that extent, lose their sense of community.

Dinner parties do not, of course, feature processed food from packets. Of course not: that would be cheating. Like expensive restaurant meals, conventional dinner-party menus in Britain are relics of the Frenchification of middle-class British food, dating from Victorian times. 'Restaurant', 'menu', 'hors d'oeuvre', 'entrée' and 'dessert' are all French words. The host of a hundred years ago despised food that looked like food. Cooking had become another French word, 'cuisine', and the way to impress your friends was to serve elaborate confections from 'recipes' with a multitude of ingredients. Cooking was turned into an 'art', to be written about and discussed like the theatre or the novel.

Dinner parties in the 1980s are simpler affairs. But look at the menu for the 'Fat' dinner party opposite. Starting with the pâté and finishing off with the cheesecake, its courses are all made from food concentrated not by machines but by hand. The pâté is fatty meat mixed with

# THE CHOICE IS YOURS

**DINNER PARTY**

| | FAT<br>1500 calories | FIT (1)<br>1500 calories | FIT (2)<br>1500 calories |
|---|---|---|---|
| | Liver pâté (3oz), white toast (1 slice) | Crudités: carrots, beetroot, peppers, tomatoes, olives, beans (total of 12oz), olive oil (3 tbsp) and lemon; wholemeal bread (2 slices) | Country soup: onions, potatoes, celery, tomatoes, cauliflower, lentils, barley, corn oil (1 tbsp); (l large bowl) wholemeal bread (2 slices) |
| | Beef Stroganoff: steak (lean) (4oz); mushrooms (1oz), onions (1oz), butter (½oz), sour cream (1oz), white rice (2oz) | Salmon trout (6oz); potatoes (boiled in skins, 6oz); broccoli (3½oz), almonds (1oz) | Jugged rabbit (4oz); onion, mushrooms (4oz); wine; oil (1 scant tbsp)<br>Butter beans (3½oz)<br>Sprouts (7oz), cheese (¾oz)<br>Carrots (6oz) |
| | Cheesecake (3½oz) | 1 pear, poached Yoghurt (2oz) | Orange syllabub (9oz) |
| | Wine (2 glasses) | Wine (3 glasses) | Wine (1 glass) |
| | Coffee, cream | Coffee, milk | Coffee, milk |
| Saturated fats<br>Sugars<br>Salt<br>Additives | HEAVY<br>HEAVY<br>MEDIUM*<br>LIGHT*** | LIGHT<br>LIGHT<br>LIGHT**<br>LIGHT | LIGHT<br>LIGHT<br>LIGHT**<br>LIGHT |
| Proteins<br>Starches<br>Fibres<br>Essential fats | RICH<br>POOR<br>POOR<br>POOR/MEDIUM | RICH<br>POOR<br>RICH<br>RICH | SUPER-RICH<br>POOR/MEDIUM<br>SUPER-RICH<br>RICH |
| Folic acid (Fo) | POOR | RICH | RICH |
| Potassium (K) | POOR | RICH | SUPER-RICH |

*if added     **if not added     ***if food home-made
Key to terms used here and on Wheels of Health: page 199.
Fit dinner party recipes: Chapter 9.

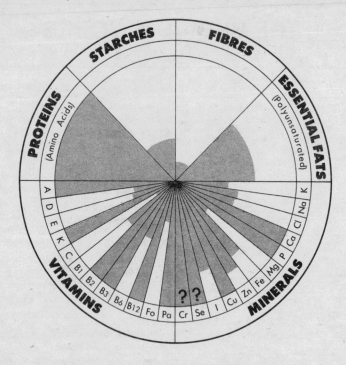

● **Fat dinner party: paté, beef stroganoff, cheesecake, wine.** There's plenty of nourishment in good fresh meat, like steak, but almost everything in this meal is intensely concentrated: on average there are over three calories in every gram of food, and cheesecake is packed with fats and sugars. This typical, fashionable European meal won't fill you and will make you fat. Menu: page 123.)

more fats, served piled on a puny slice of toast, with yet more fat as a spread. The entrée is meat in a cream sauce. The dessert is an elaboration of fats and sugars. And there's cream in the coffee. It's 'white' food originally devised for pale people: white bread, white rice, white sugar, 'white' coffee. After 1500 calories of a meal like this, you could still feel like half a dozen chocolate mints.

By contrast, look at the first Fit dinner party whose

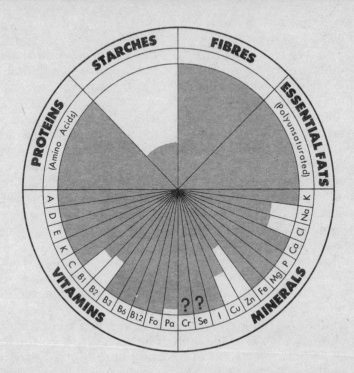

**● Fit dinner party: crudités, poached salmon trout, pears in cointreau, wine.** There's twice as much food in this meal, and room for plenty of olive oil, a sweet made with liqueur, and two glasses of wine. The abundance of vegetables, and the virtual elimination of saturated fats and processed sugars, make this a nourishing and filling feast. (Menu: page 123. Recipe: page 172.)

Wheel is above. There's another French starter – crudités – made with lots of raw and cooked vegetables, with plenty of olive oil and hunks of wholemeal bread. Altogether it's four times the weight of the pâté. The main course is fish cooked in its own juices, with potatoes and as much broccoli (steamed preferably, to remain crisp) as you like. The total of 1500 calories is made up with a simple confection of fruit with a little liqueur, and there's room for two glasses of wine, and two cups of coffee (with skimmed milk and no sugar).

You don't have to drink the wine! Like sugars, alcohol in itself is 'empty calories'. The point though, is that slimmers don't have to banish themselves to the mineral water at a dinner party.

The second Fit dinner party, whose Wheel is opposite, is even more nourishing, and even more substantial and filling; but it's still 1500 calories. It's easy to make soups with a blender, and a big bowl of thick soup is a treat. Any game animal cooked in a pot with lots of vegetables is very tasty; you don't need much of it, and some game, like rabbit, is cheap. I've found quails at £1 each: two per person is ample. And this Fit feast ends with syllabub; again, simple with a blender.

How can slimmers make a 1500 calorie meal part of a Fit day? Easy. Miss lunch. And if your dinner party is at the weekend, work up an appetite with some activity: see the 'Value of Activity' chart on page 61.

Dinner parties aren't minefields, once you know what to look for. Nor are cookbooks. The secret is to go for the cooks who prefer food to look and taste of itself, like all those listed below. Some new books have 'whole' or 'health' in the title: for example, *The Taste of Health* (BBC), Colin Spencer's *Vegetarian Wholefood Cookbook* (Granada) and Kenneth Lo's *Healthy Chinese Cooking* (Pan). Others respect the rural, peasant traditions of a country or region: for example, my own favourite, Claudia Roden's *A Book of Middle Eastern Food* (Penguin), Anne Theoharous's *Cooking the Greek Way* (Methuen), Elizabeth Cass's *Spanish Cooking* (Granada), and Arto der Haroutunian's *Complete Arab Cookery* (Granada). These are all published in paperback, as are the 'classic' writers: Arabella Boxer (*Mediterranean Cookbook*, Penguin), Jane Grigson (*Fish Cookery*, Penguin), and Elizabeth David (*Mediterranean Food*, also Penguin). Avoid or adapt dishes by these writers when they use butter, cream or sugar.

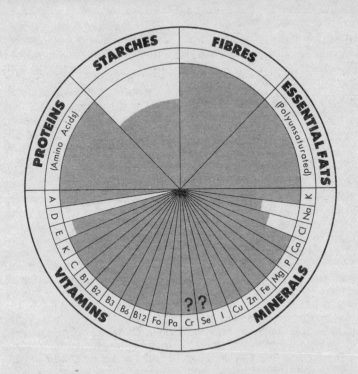

● **Fit dinner party: country soup, jugged rabbit with butter beans, syllabub, wine.** An easily prepared feast for a cold evening: lashings of thick vegetable soup, rabbit with masses of vegetables, and piquant dessert. This dinner weighs in at only one calorie per gram: very satisfying, and almost a perfectly balanced meal which is super-rich in fibres and many vitamins and minerals. (Menu: page 123.)

Fit food is for everybody, not only slimmers. You may have gained the impression that there's one kind of food for slimmers (chicken and lettuce, I was taught), another kind of food for men (a slab of meat with two veg), special food for avoiding heart attacks (low fat) or for diabetics (no sugar), and yet another type – 'health food'.

But the basic message is as simple as can be: eat plenty of whole, fresh food. This matters most at times of growth,

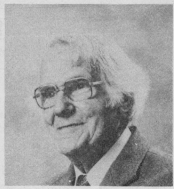

What do obesity, constipation, heart disease, some cancers, tooth decay and diabetes have in common? It was **Dr Hugh Trowell** (above) who first used the term 'Western disease' to refer to a pattern of illnesses which he saw essentially as man-made, and caused by a food supply heavy in fats and sugars, poor in fibre-rich food.

Dr Trowell worked in East Africa for thirty years, and came to realize that many of the most common causes of death and disability in Western countries are rare or even non-existent among country people in Africa.

Dr Trowell is acknowledged worldwide as the originator of the term 'dietary fibre', and he has, with Dr Denis Burkitt and, later, Dr Kenneth Heaton, edited a number of textbooks.

He is also concerned about the enthusiasm, even mania, among experts, for high-protein food, and most of all about the feeding of infants with high-protein, high-fat cows' milk. 'The human species grew up more slowly than any other primate, with the weakest breast milk' he points out. But in the last century 'we've overdone it. We've overgrown our children. If you push more than half a pint of full-fat cows' milk into a baby no good will come of it.'

In the last hundred years children have become sexually mature much younger. One result is schoolchildren with sex, not study, on their minds. And for women, he believes there is a link between fatness in infancy, early sexual maturity, and diabetes and breast cancer in later life. For good health, slow growth is best.

not only for pregnant women, but also for children, from birth to adult life. Fit food, the best food for you, slimmer or not, is also the best food for your children. The only difference is that active, growing children have big, healthy appetites – they'll often eat more than adults.

What children don't need is special concentrated food, whether this be lots of full-fat milk (concentrated in fats as well as protein), cheese (fats and proteins again), or chocolate confectionery (sweet fat). Stuffing children with concentrated foods will make them fat and will train them to prefer Fat food all their lives. If you mask the natural tastes of good food with sugars and salt, and give children confectionery as a reward, then it's hardly surprising that such a child will grow up craving sugared and salted food. Do kids who are not given sweets and chips with every-thing, crave them? Wise parents don't think so.

If you have schoolchildren, you will know that schools are no longer required to provide nourishing lunches. Officially, the standard of British food is so good that our children don't need any protection with well-spent tax-payers' money. In truth, food supplied to children is bad and getting worse. A government survey of eleven- to fourteen-year-olds, completed in 1983, showed that their diet is swamped by the Fat Five; colas, cakes, chocolate, confectionery and chips. The survey was suppressed and never published, so it's unofficial.

Look after your children. Adapt the sandwich bar ideas in chapter 1, for packed lunches. Check the policy of your local district education and health authorities. Your child-ren have a right to Fit food at school. Demand it. The same applies to other institutional food, notably in hospitals. Many in-patients and most hospitalized old people are suffering from malnutrition. Insist on your rights and those of your family. If you don't get satisfaction write to your local MP. Make a fuss. It works●

# BLIND SCIENCE

Did you hear about the man who discovered the cure for the common cold? No? Well, what happened was that word got out to the trade. So one night, there was a knock, knock, knock, and he opened his front door – who should be standing there but three burly men from the hanky trade. 'Could we have a word?' said one of the burly men. 'We'd like to make you an offer'. And that's why you never

# PROTEINS: TOO MUCH!

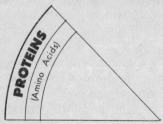

**PROTEINS**
(Amino Acids)

Proteins build the body. Like fats and sugars, there is really no such thing as 'protein': the correct term is 'proteins', which are made up of combinations of amino acids, just as fats are made up of combinations of fatty acids.

Some amino acids can be made by the body. Others must come from proteins in the diet. These are the essential amino acids, so-called because, like essential fats, vitamins and minerals, we cannot do without them in food.

Stop somebody in the street and ask them about protein and you'll probably be told that protein makes babies bonny and bouncy, and kids big and strong. Therefore, it's common knowledge that protein is a Good Thing, and that foods high in protein are good for you. Protein supplements are sold in 'health food' shops along with vitamin and mineral pills. Weightlifters and bodybuilders are said to swear by steak and eggs (both high in protein). And animal protein (from meat and dairy products) has been reckoned to be superior to vegetable protein.

What truth is there in these ideas about protein? And what is it, anyway?

Amino acids are found in different combinations within protein in food. Biochemists at the turn of the century calculated that rats grew better on amino acid combinations as found in foods of animal origin. This finding excited social reformers concerned about the stunting of the urban working class, common at that time. Practical politicians realized that feeble young men and women were not much use in wartime, so promotion of 'first-

heard of the cure for the common cold.

Pure fiction, of course. But when I say that as a rule, the reason why people get fat is simple – fats, sugars and inactivity – and the way to get fit is simple – plenty of whole, fresh food, and fresh air – I am reminded of the man in the joke.

For obesity experts are very keen on the idea that the cause and cure of flab is very, very complicated. Take this,

class' animal protein became government policy. This is why Britain today, half a century and more later, grossly over-produces cows' milk, why full-fat milk is subsidized, and why dried cows' milk, glutting Western countries, is shipped out to developing countries in the name of progress.

It is true that concentrated food, high in protein and heavy in fats, can protect the lives of starving people. Likewise, empty energy from sugars can revive a dying child. This is food used, in effect, as medi-cine, but children in the poorest countries need more than energy, and are short not just of proteins.

Because governments every-where push protein, and encourage its growth and manufacture, everybody in the West consumes more than they need. You may have noticed, in this book, that every Wheel of Health, Fat or Fit, shows a full 'proteins' segment.

The big difference between Fat and Fit food is that Fit food includes a lot more vegetable proteins (from bread, wheat, rice, beans, pulses, for instance), leaves out a lot of animal proteins, heavy in satu-rated fats, and favours other animal proteins (notably from fish), rich in essential fats.

There is no disadvantage in this. It is now well-known that animal proteins are in no way superior to well-combined vegetable proteins. In any case, it looks as if we in the West eat too many proteins from animal sources. A diet high in proteins and saturated fats causes premature growth and puberty, and may lead to premature degeneration in later life.

The idea that Big is Beautiful is, in any case, rather old-fashioned. The outstanding example of a nation whose physical growth has been accelerated on a high-protein diet, is the USA. You will have seen photographs of great, beefy American soldiers towering over small, slim peasants, at the time of the Vietnam War. And who won?

for instance, from an official advisory report. 'An intake of food in excess of requirements is usually regarded as a failure of appetite control. This may result from social, psychological, metabolic or genetic factors, operating through a final common pathway, the hypothalamus.' Or this introduction to a textbook on obesity: 'Any discussion of etiology or treatment at the present time, must involve social and psychological considerations as well as the input

# FAT FOODS

This book is full of good news about good food. Here is the news about bad food, the stuff that makes you fat. If you want to read a whole book on the subject, try *The Food Scandal* which I wrote together with Caroline Walker (see page 200).

The stuff that makes you fat ('food' really is too polite a word to use) contains calories (energy) but little or no nourishment. It's as simple as that. More and more of the Western food supply – the food manufactured and supplied to the shops – is highly processed and lacking in nourishment.

This isn't because manufacturers want to poison the population, it's just that whole, fresh food, rich in nourishment, doesn't keep. Dead food is a better commodity: it can stay on the shelf months before – or after – you buy it.

The chief dead foods are saturated fats and processed ('refined') sugars. If you want to move from Fat to Fit, avoid all saturated fats, including full-fat milk and butter, as well as fatty meat and meat products. All fats labelled 'hydrogenated' are artificially saturated.

Processed sugars come in all sorts of guises. On a food label 'sugar', 'sucrose', 'glucose', 'fructose', 'maltose', 'dextrose' are all processed sugars, as are all syrups.

Both sugars and salt also function as preservatives in food, so both are abused by manufacturers. Average salt (sodium or Na) consumption is around ten times what the body needs. Both processed sugars and salt have the effect of making you hungry or thirsty for more.

The sweet or salty product is further disguised by chemical additives, which fool you into thinking that Fat food is good food. The real truth is that it supplies little or nothing but calories.

from neurophysiology, biochemistry, pharmacology and other descriptions'. That should keep a hundred university departments of bariatrics (academic jargon for the study of flab) going indefinitely.

There is no vested interest in good health. Generally speaking, people in the Fat business, whether academics, fat-farmkeepers, metabolic druggists, no-cal cocktail mixers, or slimming moguls, have an interest in Fat people. After all, if we all got Fit, bariatricians would go bust. Which reminds me of the one about the man who invented the everlasting light bulb. But that's another story . . .

Of course there *are* people in government, science and industry who are worried about the effect the food supply has on the national health, but enormous economic imperatives work against them. For example, the total advertising budget of the sugar and chocolate confectionery industry in Britain (1985 figure) is over £400,000,000 a year. The budget of the government-funded Health Education Council, for food and health, is £500,000 a year: a very small morsel of the yearly £312,000,000 the government gets from tax on confectionery.

One very obvious approach to the question of why people gain fat, and what to do about it, is to look at those peoples in the world who don't get fat, and to consider their styles of life. Another approach is to consider what people – and animals – who get fat have in common. Essentially these approaches are simple. For example, Chinese people in mainland China as a rule do not get fat. They eat lots of rice and vegetables, not much fats, little sugars, and walk a lot, or else ride bicycles. But I have yet to find any discussion in a textbook or learned journal on obesity, looking at relevant differences between us and the Chinese. Considering there are 1,000,000,000 Chinese people, this is a remarkable omission. One day, perhaps Western knowledge will match Chinese wisdom●

## SPEEDING YOURSELF UP

Until recently the dieting books typically said or implied that if you want to lose fat, exercise won't get you anywhere. One book that I read in my calorie-cutting days said that any good that might be done by half an hour's

# HOW TO GET FIT

This table shows how long it will take you to gain the extra energy you need to move from Fat to Fit. The left-hand column applies to all able-bodied people, men as well as women. The figures show how much time it will take you to reach the target of an extra 300 calories a day (400 or so for a man) in different activities and sports. For explanation of the 'training effect' see 'Speeding Yourself Up' (page 133).

Also see Chapter 10, and the chart on page 61.

| Activity | Value above 'baseline' cals/min | Time needed to reach extra calories target | Time needed to reach target after the training effect |
|---|---|---|---|
| Sleeping | (below) | | |
| Resting | (below) | | |
| Sitting | (below) | | |
| Eating | (below) | | |
| Standing | 0.0 | infinity | |
| Writing | 0.1 – 0.2 | 25 – 50 hours | |
| Driving* | 0.5 – 0.7 | 7 – 10 hours | |
| Mending | 0.5 – 0.7 | 7 – 10 hours | |
| Cooking | 1.0 – 1.2 | 4 – 5 hours | |
| Love-making* | 1.0 – 5.0 | 1 – 5 hours | |
| Shopping | 1.5 – 4.0 | 75 – 200 minutes | |
| Walking | 1.5 – 5.0 | 60 – 200 minutes | 40 – 130 minutes |
| Cleaning | 1.5 – 6.0 | 50 – 200 minutes | |
| Gardening | 1.5 – 6.0 | 50 – 200 minutes | |
| Dancing* | 1.5 – 6.0 | 50 – 200 minutes | 33 – 130 minutes |
| Tennis* | 1.5 – 6.0 | 50 – 200 minutes | |
| Climbing | 2.5 – 7.0 | 43 – 120 minutes | |
| Cycling | 2.5 – 8.0 | 37 – 120 minutes | 25 – 80 minutes** |
| Swimming* | 4.5 – 10.0 | 30 – 66 minutes | 20 – 45 minutes** |
| Running | 4.5 – 14.0 | 22 – 66 minutes | 15 – 45 minutes** |

* when in motion   ** takes effect only after 30 minutes of continuous exercise

vigorous cycling would be immediately undone by one iced cup-cake. Another said that the fabled run of Pheidippides from Marathon to Athens (in the legend he died on arrival) was worth a mere 2500 calories, which is equivalent to less than a pound of fat. And much good it did him! For a slimmer the message was clear enough. If you want to exercise, feel free. But if you want to lose fat, stop stuffing yourself. I believed the books and discounted the fact that the one time in my life when I didn't tend to put on weight, was when I enjoyed sport at school. A mystery, I thought to myself. Nothing to do with exercise. That's what the experts say.

As we showed in *Dieting Makes You Fat*, a key fact ignored by the dieting books is that calorie-cutting slows you down. When you eat a lot less, you are in effect training your body to endure famine or starvation. The result is that your rate of metabolism slows down, not just when you are dieting, but at all times.

The reverse side of this coin is that exercise *of certain types* speeds you up, not just during the exercise, but afterwards. When you are fit enough to sustain a steady rate of exercise for half an hour or more, the 'training effect' adapts your body, so that your overall metabolic rate – which simply means the rate at which your body uses energy – speeds up. This 'training effect' is a continuous process. Unlike a car, you can steadily increase the engine capacity of your body.

You can observe this for yourself. If you go for a long, vigorous walk (or a run, if you are already Fit) you will feel warmer for some time afterwards. If you exercise regularly, you will notice that offices and other people's homes can be uncomfortably hot – not for them, but for you. On cold days you will be less likely to wear an overcoat than other people in the street; you want less bedding than an inactive partner. This extra body heat *means* that you have become more metabolically active.

It's only so-called 'aerobic' exercise that has this all-day training effect. 'Aerobic' simply means 'with air'. Aerobic exercise is now taken to mean vigorous exercise which an able-bodied person can sustain, just short of breathlessness, for long periods of time. For an unfit person, brisk walking is aerobic. As you become Fit and Superfit, you speed up, so that jogging and then running are aerobic. Likewise, cycling, dancing and swimming are aerobic exercise, and will speed you up at all times, once you are Fit enough to keep going for half an hour or more *without slowing down or stopping*●

# WHAT'S YOUR SPORT?

According to a recent survey, Britain is bottom of the European league as far as sports participation is concerned. Less and less people are involved in outdoor games. And girls dislike joining in sport more than boys do. After school few women take regular, formal exercise of any kind. Women are much more self-conscious than men about running around in public half-undressed. Men don't help here: women playing sport get leered at, and women running alone get jeered at. On my local canal towpath, 'fly fisherman' has a whole new meaning.

Below are listed a dozen sports; plus, there are a couple of rows for you to fill in any sport not on the list. Don't just tick the boxes. Write: 'Love', 'Like', 'OK', 'Dislike' or 'Hate' instead.

First, though, think back to how you felt about sport at school.

Compared with other people I know, I would say my feeling about sport at school was:

|  | Hated | Disliked | OK | Liked | Loved |
|---|---|---|---|---|---|
| School sport |  |  |  |  |  |

I would rate my level of exercise and sport now, and how I feel about it, as follows:

|  | Daily | Weekly | Monthly | Yearly | Never |
|---|---|---|---|---|---|
| 'Aerobics'/keep-fit |  |  |  |  |  |
| Body-building |  |  |  |  |  |
| Cycling (leisure) |  |  |  |  |  |
| Gym |  |  |  |  |  |
| Judo/Martial arts |  |  |  |  |  |
| Running |  |  |  |  |  |
| Sailing (racing) |  |  |  |  |  |
| Skating |  |  |  |  |  |
| Ski-ing |  |  |  |  |  |
| Squash |  |  |  |  |  |
| Swimming |  |  |  |  |  |
| Tennis (match) |  |  |  |  |  |
| Other (name) |  |  |  |  |  |
| Other (name) |  |  |  |  |  |

# FAT TO FIT

## 8

# A WHOLE FRESH DAY

**So how does it all add up? Here is a day of typical Fat food in all its horror, and two days of whole fresh Fit food in all its glory ● Yes, you can buy Fit food anywhere. But what about the cost and convenience? How to find Fit food if you don't eat meat or don't have any money ● Some advice from Caroline Walker, adviser to the BBC TV 'Food and Health Campaign'. And all you need to know: twelve tips on switching from FAT TO FIT eating, plus a shopping swapping list ● And have fun with the FAT TO FIT quizzes**

What are you eating today? And what do your family and friends eat? Here's a typical day's eating, made up of foods readily available in the shops, as consumed by millions. Breakfast: cornflakes, toast and marmalade, coffee with a sugar. Lunch from a sandwich bar: bacon sandwich and crisps, a no-cal drink to cut calories, and a small bar of chocolate confectionery for a snack. Supper: grilled chop to cut down the fat, with chips and peas, followed by a bite of apple crumble. Sounds familiar? The 'menu' for the day is shown on page 139. It's made up of the Fat meals shown on pages 24, 36 and 52, plus a little Fit snack – an orange.

This is typical British food. Surveys show that just over two fifths of the calories in the food supply come from fats, of which a half are saturated. The same is true of this Fat day. And notice that the bacon and the chop are both grilled in their own fat: had they been fried, over half this day's calories would have come from fats.

It's also known that about one fifth of the calories in the food supply come from processed, added sugars (most of which is 'hidden' in processed food). Almost the same is true of this Fat day, with about one sixth of its calories coming from processed sugars.

You might have supposed that ready-to-eat breakfast cereals and white bread 'fortified' with a few vitamins and minerals, plus an orange, would 'make all the difference' to the quality of your food. Sorry. Not true. Have a look at the Fat Wheel of Health, overleaf on page 140. Like the national food supply (page 97, and on the back cover) a day of Fat food falls short of most of the nutrients you need for good health. With less meat and more sweet food it would be worse still.

The important thing for slimmers, though, is that Fat food doesn't fill you up. This is mainly because highly processed food is concentrated by machines. Again, look at the 'menu' opposite. Excluding cups of tea or coffee or water to drink, the Fat food for a day weighs in at a little over two pounds in weight, or 1000 grams. That is to say, typical Fat food contains two calories for every gram.

By contrast, Fit food is over twice as bulky, and therefore fills you up. When we came to add up the weight of the two days of Fit food, we were fascinated to find that they weighed exactly the same: over five pounds, or 2350 grams. This means that Fit food contains less than one calorie for every gram in weight.

The first Fit day is made up of tomatoes on toast, with yoghurt and fruit for breakfast (page 39); sardines and salads with bread for lunch (page 27); and liver and vege-

# THE CHOICE IS YOURS

## A DAY'S MEALS

|  | FAT<br>2000 calories | FIT (1)<br>2000 calories | FIT (2)<br>2000 calories |
|---|---|---|---|
| Cereals | White bread<br>(3 slices)<br>Cornflakes (1 oz) | Wholemeal bread<br>(4 slices)<br>Noodles (2 oz) | Wholemeal bread<br>(1 slice)<br>Brown rice (3½ oz)<br>Oatmeal (2 oz) |
| Vegetables | Chips (3 oz)<br>Peas (2 oz) | Potatoes (3½ oz)<br>Beans (7 oz)<br>Carrots (3½ oz)<br>Onions (3½ oz)<br>Tomatoes (8 oz)<br>Cauliflower<br>(3½ oz)<br>Broccoli (3½ oz)<br>Mushrooms (2 oz)<br>Celery (2 oz) | Potato (7 oz)<br>Carrots (3½ oz)<br>Leeks (3½ oz)<br>Onions (7 oz)<br>Tomatoes (7 oz)<br>Parsnip (3½ oz)<br>Sweetcorn (2 oz)<br>Mushrooms<br>(3½ oz)<br>Pepper (2 oz)<br>Lettuce (3½ oz) |
| Fruit | Orange (3½ oz) | Banana (3 oz)<br>Pear (3½ oz)<br>Apricot (6 oz)<br>Peach (3½ oz)<br>Strawberries<br>(3½ oz)<br>Raisins (½ oz) | Banana (4½ oz)<br>Pear (6 oz)<br>Apricot (2 oz)<br>Peach (3½ oz)<br>Apple (2 oz)<br>Dates (1 oz)<br>Grapes (6 oz) |
| Meat, Fish | Chop (5 oz)<br>Bacon (1½ oz) | Liver (5½ oz)<br>Sardines (3½ oz) | Chicken (3½ oz) |
| Milk, dairy | Fat milk (6 oz)<br>Butter (½ oz) | Skim milk (1½ oz)<br>Yoghurt (8½ oz) | Skim milk (6 oz)<br>Yoghurt (3 oz)<br>Butter (¼ oz) |
| Fats, sugars | Corn oil (10 g)<br>Crisps (1 oz)<br>Crumble (2 oz)<br>Choc (1½ oz)<br>Marmalade (¾ oz)<br>Sugar (½ oz) | Corn oil (24 g)<br>Salad dressing<br>(½ oz) | Corn oil (17 g) |
| Other | No-cal (4 oz)<br>Custard (1 oz) | Wine (½ glass) | Almonds (½ oz) |
| Weight | 2 lb 4 oz (1000 g) | 5 lb 4 oz (2350 g) | 5 lb 4 oz (2350 g) |

Note: 3½ oz is 100 grams

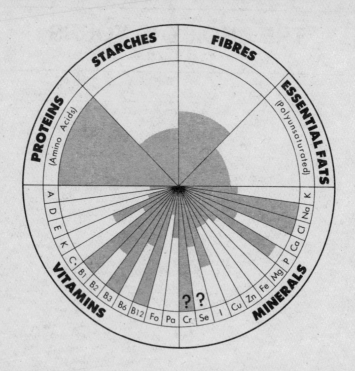

● **Fat day: processed cereal plus fats and sugars** (breakfast, page 36); **bacon and processed snacks** (lunch, page 24); **chop, chips and peas, and crumble** (supper, page 52). This typical day's food, as eaten by millions, adds up to 2000 calories. Like the national average food supply (pages 97 and 183) it's rich in protein, heavy in fats and sugars, poor in overall nourishment.

table stir-fry followed by fruit salad for supper (page 55). You can buy every single one of the items for this Fit day in one well-stocked supermarket (fruit in season of course).

Nearly an ounce of corn oil is used to cook this day's food, but total fats are down compared with the Fat day (thirty-three per cent of total calories compared with forty-three per cent); and saturated fats are way down (six and a

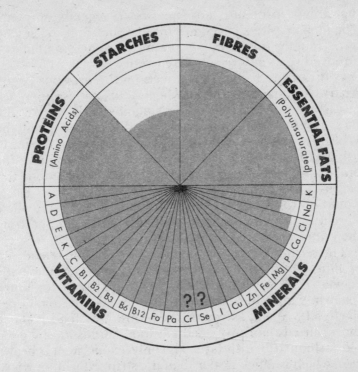

● **Fit day: savoury toast with fruit** (breakfast, page 39); **fish and fresh vegetables** (lunch, page 27); **liver and vegetable stir-fry, noodles, and fool salad** (supper, page 55). Also 2000 calories, this day's food is twice as filling as the Fat day. The wholegrain bread, the fresh fish and meat, and the masses of vegetables and fruit make this (starches apart) a perfectly balanced day's food.

half per cent of total calories compared with twenty per cent). All the sugars in the Fit day are from natural sources.

The sardines and the liver make this Fit day super-rich in proteins from animal sources. If you prefer, you can cut down the amount of meat and fish, and instead eat more high-quality bread, and switch to protein from vegetable sources such as beans. If you are vegetarian, you will know that animal protein is not superior to vegetable protein. The idea that we all need lots of steak and eggs to keep up our strength, is based on experiments done on animals a hundred years ago, which were wrong.

Contrast the Fat and Fit wheels on the previous pages. Apart from starches, the Fit wheel is full, and is super-rich in various nutrients including vitamins A, K, C, B2, B3, B12, and folic acid, calcium (Ca), and iron (Fe). To fill the Wheel for starches you'd need to cut out most of the meat, fish and fruit and replace them with double or more the bread and potatoes, or cereals like rice. I haven't done this because you might find the result rather dull to eat. I would go for a target of half of total calories from whole starches and whole sugars added together, emphasizing the value of seasonal fruits of all varieties.

The second Fit day, whose Wheel is opposite, is made up of muesli and fruit for breakfast (page 37); home-made vegetable soup with a baked potato, and fruit for lunch (page 69); and chicken risotto plus stewed fruit for supper (page 53). Again, as you can see, this day's food is much more varied than processed Fat food, and is mostly good old-fashioned British fare. The only 'exotic' item is brown rice, which is much tastier than the stripped white variety. In the 1980s we have the great advantage of more abundantly available vegetables and fruit: ten years ago sweetcorn, mushrooms and peppers were not always easy to find, and apricots, peaches and grapes were less available. By contrast, recently a stall in my local Portobello Road market was flogging off *papayas* by the crateload.

Guidelines for healthy eating, published in Western and Westernized countries all over the world, recommend rightly that we cut back on all fats. A reliable recommendation is that total fats be cut from forty-two per cent to thirty per cent of all calories, and that saturated fats be cut from around twenty per cent to a maximum of ten per cent of total calories. Representatives of the manufacturers of processed food often claim that any such

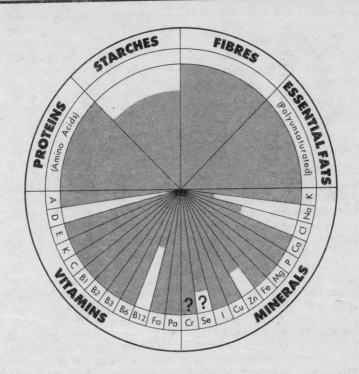

● **Fit day: muesli with fruit** (breakfast, page 37); **home-made soup, bread, jacket potato, fruit** (lunch, page 69); **chicken risotto, and stewed fruit** (supper, page 53). Another day of Fit food, so filling that it's quite difficult to make it up to 2000 calories. More bread and less fruit would fill the Wheel with starches. Low salt (Na and Cl) is no bad thing.

change would be unpalatable, unpatriotic and impossible.

Stuff and nonsense. Total fats in this second Fit day are twenty per cent or one fifth of total calories, and saturated fats four and a half per cent. The day is rich in proteins and essential fats (less so than the other Fit day) and includes rather more starches and sugars in whole form.

There is no need for any individual day's Wheel of Health to be completely full. One reason is that a number

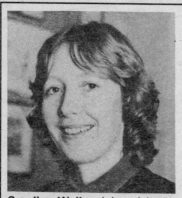

**Caroline Walker** (above) is the nutritionist who knows how to put modern knowledge about food and health across, in words that everybody can understand. She is known to government officials as 'the sock lady'. This is not because she socks it to them, but because she once invited a top-level conference to compare the amount of information on sock and sausage labels. Picking her point up, Conservative MP Jonathan Aitken has said 'we know more about what goes into a pair of socks than what goes into our food.'

She was Secretary of the working party, led by Professor Philip James, that compiled the NACNE report on dietary goals for Britain. She is a member of the Council of the Coronary Prevention Group, and works in the community in Hackney, the most deprived borough in England.

'Long ago the British population lost its agricultural roots' she says. 'People in the cities, and in the countryside, have suffered sub-standard food for many generations. What has emerged is a highly centralized food manufacturing industry, dependent on commercial fats and sugars, with chemical additives, backed by successive governments bent on a cheap-food policy at all costs.'

Co-author of *The Food Scandal*, and contributor to *Additives: Your Complete Survival Guide*, she is working on a new book, on food standards. 'Did you know that "fruit flavoured" on a packet means there's some fruit in the product, whereas "fruit flavour" means no fruit ... I call that legalized consumer fraud.'

of nutrients are stored in the body for long periods and don't need to be replenished daily.

Can you eat 2350 grams, or five pounds four ounces, of Fit food a day? It's a good question. It's a lot of food. My advice to you is have a go. If you want to get serious about it, take your scales out of the bathroom and move them into the kitchen. Stop weighing yourself, and start weighing your day's food, just for a while. It's fun to see just how much food you can tuck away.

Everybody is different. Of course small people need less food than big people, and the more active you are, as you follow the Fit plan, the bigger your natural appetite. So at first, especially if you are small, you may find that you are really full eating smaller versions of the Fit meals recommended here. That's fine, just as long as the meals really do fill you up.

Above all, don't cut down or cut out breakfast. You've seen the advertisements showing bright, smiling, active children skipping off to school after breakfast. Look after yourself the same way; treat yourself to a tasty Fit breakfast, every day●

# WHAT'S IT WORTH?

Convenient and cheap. That's what the manufacturers of highly processed food say about their products. Indeed, what else can they say? In Britain, we have been trained to prefer cheap food, but the policy which led to this wasn't just the food industry's idea. It is, after all, a pretty stupid policy. Car manufacturers don't spend all their money telling us that the cheap vehicle is the one to buy. We want value for money, but we don't usually imagine that the cheapest is best.

The cheap-food policy was invented by government, not recently, but half a century ago. At the time there was a good reason. The working population had to be made fit to fight, in a new Great War. Furthermore, Britain had to be made self-sufficient in food production, and proof against blockade by enemy ships. Therefore, people from government, science and industry worked out what the minimum food requirements were for good health, so that the country could waste not, want not, and keep the troops fighting-fit. At the same time, all available land was turned over to the most intensive possible cultivation, with the aid and support of the agri-chemical industry.

# THE DOS AND DON'TS OF FIT EATING

Is it possible to summarize the best advice about good and healthy food – the food that keeps you Fit – in two pages? Yes, it is.

## SIX DOS

**Choose plenty of whole, fresh food, and prefer food of vegetable origin.**

1. **Bread.** Eat lots more good-quality, solid wholemeal bread. Eat bread at all main meals. Eat sandwiches, not greasy pies or rolls, at lunchtime. Good-quality bread does not need fatty or sugary spreads.

2. **Potatoes, pastas, rice.** Like bread, these are not fattening in themselves. Eat lots of potatoes, preferably whole. Cut out fried potatoes and chips. Eat more rice and pastas. Brown rice is easier to cook.

3. **Vegetables, fruit.** Feast on every variety. Cook green vegetables very lightly so they stay crisp. Eat filling salads. Try beans and pulses. Enjoy fresh and dried fruit instead of fatty, sugary snacks.

4. **Meat, fish.** Healthy flesh comes from animals that live fit and healthy lives. Prefer free-range chicken. Oily fish are very good for you. So are game animals, whether expensive (venison) or cheap (rabbit).

5. **Milk, dairy products.** Without fat, dairy products are nourishing. So switch to skimmed milk, use yoghurt instead of cream, prefer low-fat or mature cheeses, cut back on butter. Three eggs a week is all right.

6. **Fats, oils.** Pure, high-quality oils – soya, sunflower, safflower, sesame, walnut, olive – are good for you, used sparingly. Use high-

After the war, nobody got around to lifting this siege mentality. People now in government, science and industry are sleepwalkers: they're not aware that they are following a policy of no relevance to the age in which we live. And that is why our food supply is Fat and cheap. On the distribution side, small uniform packages of food are cheap to make, store, shift and display. So, it will cost you under £2 a person to buy the day's Fat food shown in this

quality, unblended oils. The essential fats in fish, cereals, seeds and nuts are healthy.

## SIX DON'TS

**Avoid all highly processed foods, and processed fats and sugars most of all.**

1. **Sugars.** Added, processed sugars make you fat. They have no place in a healthy diet. Sucrose, glucose, fructose, dextrose, sugar, syrup – watch out for the names on labels. Natural sugars in fruits are fine.

2. **Fats.** Don't eat fatty meats, or processed meat products. Don't eat hard or hardened ('hydrogenated') fats and oils, or 'sweet fat' – cakes, biscuits, puddings, snacks, chocolate; fat made palatable with additives.

3. **Drinks.** Soft drinks and colas, and 'health' fruit drinks, are chiefly made of sugars and water, with additives. Always prefer whole fruit and additive-free fruit juices. Alcohol in any form has no health value.

4. **Snacks.** As a rule, the more any food is advertised on television, the worse it is for your health. Most processed snacks are made of processed sugars and/or fats. Enjoy fruit and sandwiches for snacks instead.

5. **Salt.** Whole, fresh food contains the right balance of salt, with all the vitamins and other minerals your body needs. Highly processed foods are often loaded with salt and sodium compounds. Don't add salt.

6. **Additives.** The more additives on the label, the more highly processed the food. Many additives can harm the health of vulnerable people. Get fit and healthy on additive-free whole, fresh food.

chapter. We reckoned the cost at around £1.80.

The first Fit day's food cost around £1.00, or two bus fares, more. If you chose to halve the liver and yoghurt and cut out the treat (strawberries and wine) the total would, we reckoned, be around £2.20. The second day's Fit food we costed at around £2.60, or a pint of beer more than the Fat day. You could save money on this day by leaving out lettuce and grapes, without which the food

# YOUR WEEKLY SHOPPING SWAPPING LIST

Here are two shopping baskets: the weekly food for a family of two

|  | What we eat now † |
|---|---|
| **Bread** | Mostly white. Some brown |
| **Flour** | White |
| **Cakes, biscuits** | . . . and pastries, wafers etc. |
| **Breakfast cereals** | Mostly with sugars and salt |
| **Pastas etc.** | . . . and rice (white) |
| **Meat (fresh)** | Beef, lamb, pork, bacon |
| **Meat (processed)** | Sausages, pies, canned meats |
| **Poultry** | Almost all chicken |
| **Fish** | Mostly frozen, tinned, fingers |
| **Potatoes** |  |
| **Vegetables (other, fresh)** | Mostly carrots, onion, cabbage |
| **Vegetables (processed)** | Tinned, frozen beans, peas, chips |
| **Fruit (fresh)** | Mostly apples, oranges, bananas |
| **Fruit (processed)** | Tinned and frozen |
| **Milk** | Almost all full-fat |
| **Cheese** | Mostly hard cheeses |
| **Butter** | Mostly salted |
| **Eggs** |  |
| **Fats** | Mostly soft margarines and lard |
| **Oils** | Blended vegetable oils |
| **Sugar (packets)** | Almost all white |
| **Jams, preserves** | . . . and marmalade, pickles |
| **Sweets, confectionery** | Including chocolate, bars |
| **Dried fruit, nuts** | With preservatives and salt |

† Household Food Consumption and Expenditure 1984 (MAFF/HMSO 1986)

comes in at about £2.00.

If you are broke, and make some careful choices, Fit food *can* be cheaper than Fat food. Many people now are choosing not to eat meat because they know they can get equivalent nourishment from whole cereals, beans, and lentils. And it's true that you can eat very good vegetarian food and pay £1.50 or less a day for food. What you also have to do, is take care buying and preparing food. That's

adults and two children. The list on the left shows the British 'national average' basket. The list on the right shows just how easy it is to change to a Fit basket. The foods marked with a star (*) are top Fit foods. The foods marked with a blob (•) are Fat foods.

| | What to do | The Fit shopping basket | |
|---|---|---|---|
| 6¾ lb | more, switch | All wholemeal | 13 lb* |
| 1¼ lb | switch | Wholemeal, brown | 1¼ lb |
| 2½ lb | less, switch | Low fats and sugars | 1 lb |
| ¾ lb | switch | Muesli, no sugars, whole grain | ¾ lb* |
| ¼ lb | switch | Wholegrain | ¼ lb* |
| 4½ lb | less, switch | Lean meat only, more variety | 3½ lb |
| 2¼ lb | cut out | High quality delicatessen | ¼ lb |
| 1½ lb | more | More variety | 2¼ lb |
| 1 lb | much more | Fresh, every variety | 4½ lb |
| 8¼ lb | more | New preferably in season | 12½ lb |
| 5 lb | much more | More variety | 12 lb* |
| 3 lb | cut out | Frozen in winter. Dried beans | 1 lb* |
| 3½ lb | much more | More variety | 9 lb* |
| 1½ lb | cut out | | |
| 13½ pt | switch | Semi-skimmed or skimmed | 13½ pt |
| ¾ lb | switch | Prefer soft cheeses | ¾ lb |
| ¾ lb | less | Prefer unsalted | ½ lb• |
| 14 | less | | 12 |
| 1½ lb | less, switch | 'High in polyunsaturates' margarine | ¾ lb |
| ¼ lb | more, switch | High polyunsaturated and olive oil | ¾ lb |
| 2½ lb | cut out | Brown is no better | ½ lb• |
| ½ lb | less | | ¼ lb |
| 1½ lb | cut out | | ¼–½ lb• |
| ¼ lb | more, switch | High quality, no salt (nuts) | ¾ lb* |

\* More if you like    • Better still, cut out altogether

time well spent whether you are poor or rich.

Put a higher value on your food. Enjoy talking about it, selecting it, preparing it. Allow yourself to enjoy walking to the shops, and picking and choosing the best produce. If you have to save pennies, save them on petrol. Feed your car less, feed yourself more. For yes, FAT TO FIT also has the answer to the world energy crisis, which is: smaller-capacity engines, bigger-capacity people●

# WHAT DO YOU THINK?

Do you enjoy filling in questionnaires about yourself? I do, unless my answers are liable to lead to a bigger income tax bill, or be used in evidence against me.

Every chapter of FAT TO FIT has included a questionnaire about yourself for you to fill in. I hope you've kept copies, as a record of who you were when you decided to move from Fat to Fit. The book is designed as a kit as well as a guide, to use as it suits you personally.

The idea has been to answer the questions without thinking about what the answer *should* be. If you bring a mood of self-consciousness into your answers, you'll lose sight of what the questions are all about, which is to allow you to see who you are at one point in time.

For example, on page 32 I suggest that you rate your general mood 'Great', 'Good', 'OK', 'Bad' or 'Awful'. Now, everybody knows that they *shouldn't* feel awful. But if you do, allow yourself to say so.

On page 64 I ask you about everyday activity and exercise. How do you compare with other people? If your picture is that people you know leap around more than you, put down 'Inactive' as your self-assessment. And so on, with all the questionnaires in the book. Tell it like it is.

This is where the following pages come in handy. They repeat the first three questionnaires. Save them up until you're three or so months into the FAT TO FIT plan, answer the questions – and see if there are any changes. The idea, of course, is not to look back and check to see what you saw three months ago before answering. This is part of the process: be where you are, not where you were or where you think you should be.

If you have access to a photocopier, you can use FAT TO FIT for as long as you like, as the means to chart your changes. Take copies of the questionnaires, stick the copies into a diary and continue to answer the questions every three months or so. If you don't have a photocopier, keep my

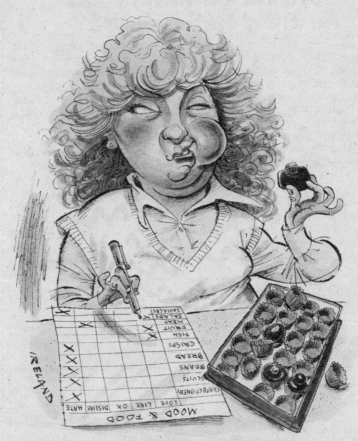

publisher happy: rip this copy up and buy another one.

FAT TO FIT is not just about losing excess fat. You may find, as you enjoy plenty of good food and fresh air, that you're less bothered about overweight. Fine. You may discover a new slim you, or you may become healthier or happier without much change in shape. That's fine too. If you transform the quality of your food and recover your lost activity, you *will* lose fat, in time. You will also gain pleasure●

# CHECK YOURSELF OUT: HOW HAS IT GONE?

In Chapter one there's a set of questions inviting you to measure yourself and record some of your feelings about yourself, your fitness and your health. Here they are again. Don't look back. Rather, now that you are on the way from Fat to Fit, fill in this page and then look at the differences.

The best way to use FAT TO FIT is over a period of six months or a year, as an everyday guide to good food and activity. The three questionnaires starting on this page are designed to support you. Take copies, stick them in a diary and record your progress each month.

You may find that your weight does not change much over the months. It's more likely that your waist measurement *will* change. Pulse rate at rest is a good indication of fitness: the slower, the fitter. You will probably find that it will slow down over the months. And have your overall feelings about yourself changed?

| Age | Height | | Weight |
|-----|--------|--|--------|
| Chest | Waist | | Hips |
| Pulse rate at rest | | Blood pressure | |

Rate the following things about yourself (tick a box)

| | Great | Good | OK | Bad | Awful |
|--|-------|------|-----|-----|-------|
| Health | | | | | |
| Fitness | | | | | |
| Self-respect | | | | | |
| General mood | | | | | |
| Energy | | | | | |

# CHANGING FOOD AND CHANGING MOOD

We have a natural taste for sweet and salty foods. In nature, sweet foods are ripe, ready to eat, and safe. The natural taste for salt is probably because sodium is fairly hard to find in nature – which is why bread has always been made with salt. But food manufacturers exploit these tastes, which can become cravings. Anybody who has been brought up on typical Western food, as supplied in Britain and America, will find that foods without added sugars and salt taste insipid.

But, after a few months on the FAT TO FIT plan, you will probably have kicked the sugars and salt habit. If you have, and now enjoy whole fresh foods that taste of themselves, you'll be interested to fill this questionnaire in and compare your feelings about different types of food with the answers you gave on page 48. If your answers haven't changed much, that will be either because you were already accustomed to good food, or because you find the sugars and salt habits hard to break. It you have access to a copying machine, take extra copies of this page and keep a record over the months.

| | Love | Like | OK | Dislike | Hate |
|---|---|---|---|---|---|
| Beans | | | | | |
| Biscuits | | | | | |
| Bread | | | | | |
| Confectionery | | | | | |
| Crisps | | | | | |
| Fish | | | | | |
| Fruit | | | | | |
| Meat | | | | | |
| Salad | | | | | |
| Sausages | | | | | |
| Soft Drinks | | | | | |
| Vegetables | | | | | |

# RECOVERING YOUR ACTION

If you've followed the FAT TO FIT plan, you'll have become a lot more aware of where the action is in your own life, and how you have recovered your lost activity in ways that suit you. You will also have noticed just how often we are discouraged from being active, most of all by using cars, but also by little things like electric typewriters, and big things like new roads built without pavements.

Chapter ten, 'The Action Plan', is specially designed to allow you to plan your activity over a whole week. And on page 64 there was a questionnaire which rated your initial level of activity. Here it is again for you to check the changes. Now that you're moving from Fat to Fit, how do you rate your activity compared with other people? And how much time have you recovered for activity and exercise? If you have access to a copying machine, take extra copies of this page and keep a record over the months.

Compared with other people I know, I would say I am

| Very active | Average | Inactive |
|---|---|---|
| | | |

On an average sort of day the amount of time I take in activity is

| Minutes | none | 1–10 | 10–30 | 30–60 | 60 plus |
|---|---|---|---|---|---|
| Cooking | | | | | |
| Cycling | | | | | |
| Dancing | | | | | |
| Driving | | | | | |
| Gardening | | | | | |
| Housework | | | | | |
| Running | | | | | |
| Shopping | | | | | |
| Swimming | | | | | |
| Walking | | | | | |
| Other (name) | | | | | |
| Other (name) | | | | | |

# FAT ⊚ FIT

## ⑨

# THE EATING PLAN

**B**reakfast, lunch, snacks, supper, dinner party: now you know the secret of Fit meals and how to combine them for a day ● Here's your plan for Fit meals for a week, for all the seasons of the year ● What if you are vegetarian? And what if you are a small eater? Here are the answers ● And here, too, are the secrets of how to find take-away and restaurant meals that will help you lose that excess fat ● Plus recipes for packed lunches and picnics

Everybody is different. Every writer and every reader of books on foods, fitness and health has to respect that. By now you will have looked through lots of Fat and Fit meals for all times of the day, and all seasons. I think our featured Fit meals are delicious, but you may have other ideas. Lots of people don't eat meat, for instance. Others don't like porridge or muesli. Suit yourself, but whatever your taste, stick to whole, fresh food, and prefer food of vegetable origin. Eat lots of wholegrain cereal, and every variety of vegetable and fruit.

Most meals in FAT TO FIT are worked out to add up to a maximum of 2000 calories a day. This is the amount of energy an 'average' woman needs and uses every day. So, as you will have read, once you get used to enjoying another 300 calories of activity every day, you can eat 2000 calories a day, and gradually lose fat.

However, if you are a woman below average height – 5 ft 4 in (1 .66m) or less, say – or if you have a small build, or if you are over forty years old and not specially active, it is probable that you use less than 2000 calories a day. And if you are a veteran of calorie-cutting diet régimes, it is very likely that these will have slowed your metabolic rate right down, and replaced lean tissue with flab.

Have a look at the meals on the following pages, arranged day by day for a week. On some days you may think to yourself, 'goodness, I couldn't eat all that in a day'. If you have become accustomed to eating typical Western food, heavy in machine-made concentrates, the sheer size of good food on the plate may amaze you. Small, lean, country people in the East pile down great bowls of rice and vegetables, so pick a day's food from the week's recipes on the following pages, and see how it goes. Trust your body: if you feel full, that's fine, but if you feel sleepy after a main meal, it is probably too large for you.

In that case, all you have to do is cut down the amounts of ingredients in the meals, in proportion. But don't cut out breakfast! Try Tuesday's choice, which adds up to 1500 calories. But don't go hungry. It takes maybe a month, perhaps two months, fully to enjoy good food if you've been used to fatty, sugary, salty stuff. If you feel happier on 1500 calories a day, or 1800 (see Thursday) that's fine.

Most of this week's food is easily adapted if you are a vegetarian, and Thursday's food is totally vegetarian. Personally, I wouldn't find it hard to cut out 'red' meat altogether, but I would like to keep offals, and would miss fish greatly. There is such a marvellous variety of tasty fish and seafood in the shops now.

Every day's meals, apart from the feast day, are based on portions for one person, so you can compare the value of each meal. You'll see that they are not the usual stingy,

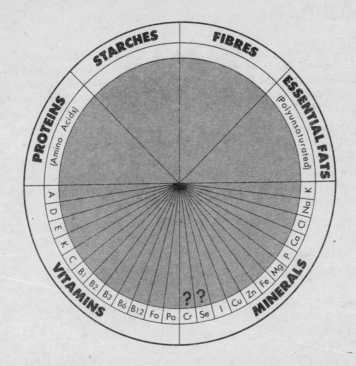

● **Fit meals for a week.** Eat well for a week, and your Wheel of Health will be completely full. This shows a genuinely balanced diet. It supplies plenty of starches, fibres and essential fats, as well as proteins. It is rich in vitamins like B₆, B₁₂ and folic acid, as well as the familiar vitamin C; and all the minerals and trace elements are included. The Eating Plan should help achieve all this.

calorie-cutting slimmers' meals, to be eaten alone. Enjoy them with your family. Each breakfast menu includes one cup of tea with milk.

The fully Fit Wheel of Health on this page illustrates journey's end for everybody who has decided to follow the FAT TO FIT plan. It's not difficult to fill your Wheel, once you decide to put a high value on the food you eat, and to enjoy everyday activity●

# MONDAY

If you like meat, and have an office job, here's a day's Fit choices for you: muesli and fruit for breakfast (see page 35); a takeaway of fish, salads and fruit for lunch (page 23); and chicken risotto followed by fruit for supper (page 51). Once you've put activity back into your life, this 2000 calories will fill you up and help make you Fit.

## Breakfast
400 calories

Muesli doesn't have to come out of packets. It was originally a do-it-yourself affair, and mixing your own gives a breakfast Fit for your own taste. Try this to start with and then experiment, changing the base to include other cereals, adding fresh fruit, a few nuts and yoghurt.

### Muesli
*50g (2oz) rolled oats*
*40g (1½oz) dried fruit*
*1 fresh peach chopped*
*100ml (3½fl oz) skimmed milk*

Mix and munch. For a drink take 1 cup of tea with skimmed milk.

## Lunch
700 calories

So often, slimmers who spend their weekdays working, skip lunch then sneak out for a chocolate snack or a bun from the tea lady. It's normal to want to eat lunch. Encourage your appetite: walk vigorously to your local sandwich bar, salad bar or supermarket. Here's an example of the kind of Fit lunch you should easily find there.

### Sardine 'n' Salad Lunch
*100g (3½oz) canned sardines with the oil drained*
*100g (3½oz) potato salad in vinaigrette*
*350g (12oz) bean and vegetable salad in vinaigrette*
*1 large wholemeal roll*
*1 peach, 2 apricots*

By choosing carefully you can buy a Fit lunch at any decent take-away or shop. Pick wholemeal rolls, pitta and salads dressed in good oils and lemon, rather than greasy mayonnaise. Drain oil from fish, and cut off skin and fat from poultry and meat, if preferred.

## Supper
900 calories

Rissotto is an ideal Fit meal. It's also a smart way to finish off the Sunday chicken. This recipe uses brown rice for its flavour. It also contains more fibre, vitamins and minerals than the stripped, white variety. Brown rice is easy to find in well-stocked supermarkets – but note that it takes longer to cook than the white stuff.

### Risotto
*100g (4oz) brown rice*
*1 tsp pure vegetable oil*
*1 small onion, peeled and chopped*
*1 small pepper, chopped*
*60g (2oz) sweetcorn (boiled)*
*1 tsp mild curry powder*
*garlic to taste – try half a small clove if unsure*
*100g (4oz) tomatoes canned with juice*
*10g (1/2oz) almonds*
*100g (4oz) cooked chicken*

First cook your rice. Measure the rice, pour into a colander and rinse under the cold tap as you bring 900ml (1½ pints) of water to the boil in a saucepan. Add the rice to the water, stir and cover., Allow to simmer for 30–45 minutes, then test. Brown rice has a pleasantly chewy texture when cooked, but if it's positively crunchy cook longer.

Heat the oil in a frying pan. Non-stick, or thick heavy cast-iron pans need the least oil. Add the pepper and onion to the pan, and fry for a couple of minutes. Now add the curry power and garlic and cook for a few minutes more over a gentle heat, stirring all the time. Add the tomatoes, breaking them into a pulp as they cook.

Mix in the cooked rice, sweetcorn and chicken, and heat thoroughly for about 7 minutes. Meanwhile toast the almonds under the grill, sprinkle on top of the risotto and serve with a green salad.

### Salad
*25g (1oz) lettuce, washed*
*50g (2oz) cucumber, cut into strips*
*25g (1oz) watercress, washed and yellow leaves discarded*
*Orange juice to dress*

Combine the cucumber and watercress and lettuce and sprinkle with orange juice for a refreshing salad.

For pudding finish off with a fruity Fit treat: stewed apricots, apples and pears topped with yoghurt.

# TUESDAY

Slimmers with small appetites often skip breakfast. Don't. This day's
Fit food adds up to 1500 calories. But it starts with a hearty breakfast:
yoghurt and fruit, and toast with a savoury topping (see page 35). A
clever choice of pub lunch steers you away from the grease. And in
the evening, a Fit favourite: a big dish of pasta.

## Breakfast
400 calories
Good wholemeal bread is an excellent Fit start to the day. Substitute
savoury toppings for fatty and sugary spreads.

### Savoury Toast
*2 slices of wholemeal bread (approximately 50g/2oz each)*
*2 fresh tomatoes, cut into slices*
*scant ½ tsp pure vegetable oil*

Toast the bread on both sides. Put the tomatoes on the toast, sprinkle
with oil and return to grill until ready.

### Home-made Fruit Yoghurt
*160g (6oz) carton plain yoghurt*
*1 chopped pear (or fruit to taste)*
*12g (½oz) raisins*

Mix together and you've got your own healthy fruit yoghurt.

### Drink
*1 cup of tea with skimmed milk*

## Pub Lunch
550 calories
You needn't avoid pub lunches. Look at the least processed, simpler
items on the board. A baked potato or salad platter is a good choice.
Most hot dishes of the day – meat pies, shepherd's pies – are very fatty.

A suitable Fit pub lunch might comprise a slice of lean roast beef
(50g/2oz approx.) and a green salad, with two wholemeal rolls,
accompanied by pickled onion, beetroot or gherkins. And you can allow
yourself a glass of white wine.

Ploughman's lunches can be Fit too, if you can find genuine locally-
baked fresh bread, and a tasty mature cheese. You won't want an
enormous slab of cheese if it's strong and of good quality. Camembert
and Brie are good choices. Insist on lots of onion and tomato.

## Supper

550 calories

Pasta is always a Fit choice. Like bread, the skill is in finding high-quality pasta and eating lots of it. This recipe is from Antonio Carluccio, an Italian chef working in London who loves simple, healthy cooking; it can be accompanied by a pea salad.

### Pasta with Leeks and Ham*

*75g (3oz) wholewheat pasta – spirals (fusili) go well*
*1/2 tsp olive oil*
*1 modest size leek, trimmed and finely chopped*
*50g (2oz) low-fat soft cheese*
*25ml (1fl oz) skimmed milk*
*50g (2oz) lean cooked ham*

Measure out the pasta and put the kettle on. Finely chop the leek and fry gently in the olive oil until soft. Fill a saucepan with the boiling water and add the pasta, giving it a stir. It really isn't necessary to add either salt or oil. While waiting for the pasta to cook you can get on with the sauce. Let it boil fairly fast for 12 minutes, then test. Perfectly cooked pasta is described as *al dente*, meaning it should still have a bit of a bite to it. Drain then return to the saucepan to keep warm.

Back to the sauce: add the chopped ham to the leeks. Mix the milk into the soft cheese to make a smooth cream. Add this to the pan with the ham and leeks and gently heat through, without boiling, for about 5 minutes. At this point the British style is to slap the pasta on a plate and pour the sauce on top. The Italians rather more cleverly allow for the possibility that the pasta might have to wait a while. So they add it to the sauce mixture at the end and cook the two together for a minute, making sure both are piping hot.

### Italian Pea Salad

*100g (4oz) peas, shelled weight*
*50g (2oz) fennel, finely sliced*
*50g (2oz) spring onions, finely sliced*
*1 tbsp vinaigrette made with 1 part pure vegetable oil and 3 parts wine vinegar*
*Lemon juice*
*Black pepper*

Simmer the peas until they are quite tender. Drain and place in a dish, then pour the vinaigrette over the peas. Leave to cool. When the peas are cold, mix in the fennel and spring onion and give a good dowsing with fresh lemon juice. Sprinkle with black pepper.

*Published in The Taste of Health (BBC Publications, £5.50).

# WEDNESDAY

What do you do if you've got no money, and want to eat cheap,
nourishing and slimming food at home, by yourself or with the
family? Take some tips from your grandparents' day. Here's porridge
for breakfast and a delicious salad for lunch (see page 67), then a liver
stir-fry for supper (page 51).

### Breakfast
400 calories
At three pence a bowl, porridge has to be the cheapest way to start the
day and its wealth of nutrients and fibre make it Fit for royalty. Here's a
traditional recipe using oatmeal rather than rolled oats. Overnight
soaking means this is just as quick as the instant variety. Water or fruit
juice can be substituted for the milk. Adding dried fruit to the soaking-
liquid gives a delicious sweetness.

#### Oatmeal Porridge
*50g (2oz) medium oatmeal*
*200ml (7fl oz) skimmed milk and water in a 50/50 mix*
*50g (2oz) dried raisins or other dried fruit*

Soak the oatmeal overnight in the milk and water mixture. Tip the lot
into a saucepan and bring to the boil, stirring all the time. This stirring
is essential unless you enjoy authentic, lumpy porridge. Reduce the heat
and simmer until the porridge reaches the thickness you prefer. For a
drink, take tea with skimmed milk.

### Lunch
600 calories
This meal can just as easily be enjoyed at home or packed up in a
sandwich-box and taken to work. For snacks, put by some cherries for
the afternoon.

#### Fish 'n' Bean salad
*Either 50g (2oz) canned tuna or mackerel or*
*100g (4oz) tinned crab or pilchard carefully drained of any oil or dressing*
*100g (4oz) canned kidney beans*
*100g (4oz) cooked frozen sweetcorn*
*100g (4oz) mustard cress*
*100g (4oz) cucumber*
*Scant tbsp vinaigrette made with 1 part vegetable oil and 3 parts wine vinegar*

Flake the fish and mix together with all the salad ingredients, sprinkle with vinaigrette. Eat with a large wholemeal roll and cherries for afters.

*1 large wholemeal roll*
*100g (4oz) fresh cherries*

## Supper
900 calories
Liver is wonderful value. Like other offals, it's packed with nourishment. Make a date with liver or kidneys every two weeks or so.

### Liver Stir-Fry
*100g (4oz) onion, chopped into fine strips*
*175g (5¹/₂oz) liver, cut into fine strips*
*100g (4oz) French beans, topped and tailed*
*100g (4oz) broccoli, florets broken off and stems chopped*
*100g (4oz) cauliflower, florets broken off and stem chopped*
*100g (4oz) carrot, cut into fine strips*
*50g (2oz) instant wholewheat noodles or pasta noodles (tagliatelle)*
*1 tbsp pure vegetable oil*

If you are using pasta, set it to boil for 12 minutes, drain and keep hot. Instant noodles do not need cooking, just put them in a bowl, cover with boiling water and leave for 4 minutes. Drain and keep hot.

The liver is stir-fried, a Chinese method which requires a minimum amount of oil, and a maximum of elbow grease because the cooking ingredients have to be turned frequently in the pan. Active cooking! A Chinese wok is the ideal thing to stir-fry in, but a large, preferably non-stick, frying pan will do.

Heat half of the oil in the pan and bring to a fairly high temperature. Add the onions and liver and get stirring. Cook for 3 to 5 minutes, so that the liver is only slightly pink in the middle, then push it and the onion to the side of the pan. Add a bit more oil, put the carrots and cauliflower into the pan stirring them all the time. Cook for 2 minutes, then add the beans and broccoli and continue to stir for another 3 minutes. The vegetables should be hot, but crisp. Finally, mix in your noodles and serve.

### Strawberry and Banana Fool
*100g (4oz) strawberries*
*¹/₂ banana*
*75g (3oz) yoghurt*
*¹/₂ glass white wine*

Purée all the ingredients together and chill well.

# THURSDAY

People who don't eat meat have a much better deal now. Wednesday's choices include meat as a relish; this day's meals, adding up to 1800 calories, are vegetarian. But everybody will enjoy the food: mushrooms on toast for breakfast, a filling lunch of baked potato and real soup (adapted from page 67); and home-made pizza for supper.

**Breakfast**
400 calories
The Fit way to enjoy mushrooms, potatoes and all vegetables and fruit with edible skin, is carefully washed and eaten whole, skins and all.

### Mushrooms on Toast
*100g (4oz) mushrooms, washed, dried, finely sliced*
*25ml (1fl oz) skimmed milk*
*2 slices wholemeal toast*

Finely slice the mushrooms. Put the bread on, to toast, and place the mushrooms in a pan with the milk, to simmer gently until they are soft and most of the milk has been absorbed. Then top the toast with the mushrooms. Finish your breakfast fruit in season.

**Lunch**
600 calories
If you are eating at home you can get this meal on the go and then nip out to do some shopping or collect the children.

### Vegetable Soup
*6g butter*
*100g (4oz) carrot, finely chopped*
*100g (4oz) leek, cleaned, trimmed and chopped*
*100g (4oz) parsnip, cleaned, trimmed and chopped*
*100g (4oz) canned tomatoes with juice*
*25g (1oz) parsley*
*1 slice wholemeal bread*

Melt the butter in a saucepan, sauté the leek, parsnips and carrot until soft, add the tomatoes and half a pint of water and bring to the boil. Cover the pan, leaving it to simmer for about 20 minutes. Chop the parsley, sprinkle it on the soup and serve with a hunk of wholemeal bread. Accompany with a baked potato, stuffed with onion and a few slices of mushroom left over from breakfast. Fruit to follow.

### Supper
800 calories
Making a pizza is easier than you may think. Take a tip from the French and use a scone base for simplicity.

#### *Pizza*
*50g (2oz) wholemeal flour*
*a pinch of bicarbonate of soda*
*12g (½fl oz) polyunsaturated margarine*
*25ml (1fl oz) skimmed milk*

*Sauce:*
*½ tsp of vegetable oil*
*½ a small onion, finely chopped*
*100g (4oz) tomatoes*
*a dash of tabasco (chilli) sauce*
*1 tsp either basil, oregano or sage, to taste*

*Topping:*
*1 small red pepper, cut into strips*
*½ small onion, cut into strips*
*1 tsp of capers*
*12g (½oz) mozzarella cheese, thinly sliced (optional)*

Pre-heat the oven to gas mark 5, 185°C (370°F). Mix the bicarbonate of soda into the flour thoroughly. Rub in the margarine, then mix in enough milk to form a soft dough. Roll the dough out into a circle about 15cm (6″) across. Place on an oiled baking-sheet and bake in the centre of the oven for 10 minutes.

While the base is cooking, make the sauce. Fry the onions in oil until soft, then add the tomatoes, the herb of your choice and a dash of tabasco. Cook this for 10 minutes, or until it will spread easily.

Spread the tomato sauce on the base, then top with a criss-cross lattice-work of pepper and onion, scattering capers in between. Finish with the cheese and return to the oven for about 15 minutes. Lift up the base (carefully!) and check the pizza is golden brown all over. Serve with a green salad and take advantage of the hot oven to make a cooked pudding – a big apple stuffed with 2oz of dates and baked until soft.

#### *Salad*
*100g (4oz) iceberg or cos lettuce, washed and thinly sliced*
*100g (4oz) watercress, washed and yellow leaves discarded*
*100g (4oz) chopped parsley*

Mix all the ingredients together and dress with lime juice.

# FRIDAY

More good news: a take-away supper can be part of your Fat to Fit plan. There are two secrets. First, know how to choose high quality take-aways. Second, enjoy lots of salad for lunch, like the delicious avocado and spinach mix below.

### Breakfast
400 calories
The occasional egg for breakfast can also be part of the plan. Just don't fry or scramble eggs in hard fats. Poaching or boiling are the simplest ways to enjoy an egg.

*Boiled-Egg Breakfast, soft boiled*
*1 medium egg (size 3 or 4)*
*2 slices of wholemeal bread (approximately 50g/2oz each)*
*a smear of polyunsaturated margarine (optional)*
*1 pear*

*Drink:*
*1 cup of tea with skimmed milk*

### Lunch
700 calories
A spinach salad can make a substantial lunch to eat by yourself or a light first course to share with friends.

*Spinach Salad*
*100g (4oz) spinach, thoroughly washed, dried and thinly sliced*
*100g (4oz) mushrooms, washed, wiped and cut into quarters*
*100g (4oz) avocado, peeled and sliced*
*50g (2oz) shelled walnuts*
*1 slice of wholemeal bread (approximately 50g/2oz)*
*1 tsp of oregano soaked in 1 tbsp vinaigrette*

Toast the bread thoroughly, then cut into small cubes. Mix all the vegetables together in a bowl along with the herb dressing. Scatter the toast cubes on top and tuck in. Enjoy a banana for afters.

## Supper: Take-away

It's Friday night, and you've decided to take it easy and get a take-away. You probably have plenty of choice but how can you find a Fit meal?

### Fish 'n' chips

If you have a good chippy near you, fish 'n' chips are no bad choice. White fish is very low in fat, and what it does contain is rich in the essential polyunsaturated variety. Potatoes contain proteins, fibres, and are rich in vitamin C, potassium and magnesium.

Buy from a chippy where the oil is clean and regularly changed, and is of good quality. Meat can be twice as fatty as battered fish that has been skilfully fried in very hot oil. And don't pick up the salt shaker; eat fish tasting of fish. Note too that 'vinegar' in most fish 'n' chip shops is nothing of the sort, but a dubious chemical concoction called 'non-brewed condiment'. Rely on the vinegar-bottle back home.

A six-ounce helping of haddock (or any white fish) and a four-ounce portion of chips comes to around 700 calories.

### Greek

If all the chippies around you merit a greasy-spoon award, go for a Greek take-away instead. Choose yoghurt-based dips such as tzatziki with plenty of pitta bread, rather than taramasalata. Shish kebabs are a good Fit option – the quality of meat used is generally much better than that which goes into doner kebab, and because it is grilled, little extra fat is added during cooking. A standard take-away salad of shredded cabbage or lettuce, cucumber, tomatoes, onions and olives, is highly nutritious and delicious.

A meal of tzatziki, shish kebab, pitta bread and salad will provide approximately 700 calories, with about a third of them coming from fats. By contrast, taramasalata, doner kebab, pitta and salad, gives about 1400 calories, with 60–70 per cent of them coming from fats. Disaster!

### Chinese

Chinese food is usually very low in fat and the vegetables are cooked quickly to preserve their texture and nourishment. Plenty of rice is generally provided, and meals are bulky without being high in calories. The only drawback is the high sodium content – monosodium glutamate and salt from soy sauce are almost impossible to avoid. Nevertheless, you can choose a reasonably Fit meal. Stir-fried chicken with mixed vegetables and a generous portion of rice would supply about 800 calories, with roughly 30 per cent coming from fats. Avoid fried-rice dishes, and ones which depend on a dose of sugar such as sweet and sour pork, or chop suey.

# SATURDAY

'Brunch' – breakfast and lunch combined – maybe as a welcome treat for visiting friends. Recover the lost pleasures of kidney, tomatoes, mushrooms and yes, sauté potatoes (see page 107). This 2000 calorie day is completed by an easy-to-cook dish of pork in orange. In the afternoon? Enjoy the fresh air and work up a healthy appetite.

## Brunch
700 calories
The cooked breakfast needn't be a thing of the past. By combining it with lunch you can enjoy it as part of your Fit plan.

### Kidneys, tomatoes and mushrooms
*200g (8oz) potatoes, washed and scrubbed*
*1 tbsp pure vegetable oil*
*200g (8oz) lambs' kidneys, sliced and with the gristly core removed*
*100g (4oz) fresh tomatoes*
*100g (4oz) mushrooms, washed, wiped and sliced*
*100g (4oz) frozen sweetcorn*

*Drink:*
*Tea with skimmed milk*

Boil the potatoes in their skins until they are just getting soft (approximately 15 minutes). Slice them thinly. Heat half the oil in a large frying pan and layer the potatoes over half of the pan surface.

Cook the kidneys and the tomatoes in the remaining space for 5 minutes, stirring frequently. Turn the potatoes over so that they brown on both sides, adding more oil if necessary. Now mix the mushrooms in with the kidney and tomato mixture, and cook for a few minutes more. Put the sweetcorn on to boil meanwhile, simmering for 2 minutes. Serve with a drink of fresh orange juice.

## Snack
400 calories
If you've spent your Saturday in an active way you may feel peckish. That's fine, have a healthy and satisfying snack.

### Camembert Sandwich
*2 slices of wholemeal bread (approximately 50g/2oz)*
*50g (2oz) Camembert cheese*
*2 sticks celery*
*Plus: a banana and an orange*

## Supper
900 calories

This supper is very simple to prepare: just what you need on a frantic Saturday evening. Apple juice and apple slices can be substituted for the orange juice and rind – feel free to experiment. There's a generous helping of rice to mop up the sauce, which you can reduce if you wish.

### Pork with Orange

*100g (4oz) uncooked brown rice*
*1 small onion, sliced lengthwise*
*1 small pepper, sliced lengthwise*
*1/2 tsp pure vegetable oil*
*100g (4oz) lean fillet (tenderloin) pork, thinly sliced*
*100ml (3 1/2 fl oz) orange juice*
*1/2 tbsp grated orange rind*
*1/2 tsp soy sauce*
*1/2 tsp arrowroot*
*100g (4oz) carrot, washed and sliced*
*100g (4oz) courgettes, washed and chopped*

Start the brown rice cooking as described on page 159. Put the carrots on to cook for 15 minutes as you prepare the main dish. Heat the oil in a frying pan and cook the pepper, onion and pork for a few minutes. Add the orange juice and rind and cook for 5 to 7 minutes or until the meat is cooked all the way through. Put the courgettes to cook for 5 minutes now. Reduce the heat. Combine the soy sauce and arrowroot in a cup with enough water to form a runny mixture and add this to the pan. Allow to thicken and then serve with the brown rice, carrots and courgettes.

### Apricot Syllabub

*100g (4oz) Hunza apricots, rinsed and soaked overnight.*
*75g (3oz) low-fat soft cheese*

Retain the soaking-water, which will have absorbed the rich taste of these tiny apricots. Remove the stones from the fruit and chop it coarsely. Blend together the apricots, cheese and water in liquidizer for a delicious dessert.

# SUNDAY

Lie in, read the papers, and enjoy a late summer breakfast of tinned salmon (yes, there are Fit tinned foods), with mounds of filling salads, a large wholemeal roll, plus a glass of wine (yes, just a little of what you fancy won't make you Fat) (see page 116). And complete your week with a treat: here's how to find Fit food in Eastern and Western restaurants.

### Brunch
700 calories

Celebrate your first Fit week with a leisurely brunch. If you've really got something to celebrate, substitute smoked salmon and champagne – real Fit luxury.

### *Salad I*
*60g (2½oz) tinned salmon*
*100g (4oz) boiled butter beans*
*100g (4oz) french beans, topped, tailed and chopped*
*100g (4oz) fresh tomato*
*25g (1oz) black olives*
*1 tbsp vinaigrette made with 1 part pure vegetable oil and 3 parts wine vinegar*

Mix all the ingredients together and brush with oil and lemon.

### *Salad II*
*25g (1oz) chicory, washed and sliced*
*50g (2oz) orange fresh, sliced*
*25g (1oz) watercress, washed and with yellow leaves discarded*
*25g (1oz) celery, washed and sliced*
*1 tbsp vinaigrette made as above*

Mix all the ingredients together and brush with oil and lemon.

### *Salad III*
*100g (4oz) carrots, washed and grated*
*100g (4oz) cabbage heart, grated*
*1 tbsp vinaigrette made as above*

Mix all the ingredients together and brush with oil and lemon.

Arrange the three separate salads in circles on a plate, with the salmon in the middle and eat with the wholemeal bread. Enjoy a glass (100ml/3½ fl oz) of white wine. Your good health!

## Supper: eating out

Fit restaurant meals are not hard to find. Just avoid French *haute cuisine*. Mediterranean and Eastern restaurants really serve Fit food, if you know what to look for. And – more good news – the more pasta and rice you eat, the smaller the bill.

### Indian

The Indian staple diet is cereal-based, with rice, breads, lentils and beans forming the bulk of meals. It will provide enough fibres, vitamins and minerals to fill your Wheel without an excess of fattening, artery-clogging fats. If you want to get a Fit meal in an Indian restaurant, the best choice is a pilau – a rice-based dish with vegetables or meat, but without fatty sauces. Tandoori dishes are marinaded in yoghurt and spices, brushed with a little fat and then cooked with no further fat in a clay oven. Good restaurants do not use artificial colourings in their tandooris. If you feel hard-done-by without some sort of curry, go for a mixed vegetable one. Add raita (yoghurt with cucumber, garlic and spices) or dhal (curried lentils) or nan (unleavened bread) or chapatis to your order. Avoid bhajis, samosas and puris which tend to be Fat rather than Fit.

A chicken tikka or tandoori chicken, vegetable curry, chapati, and nan will give you roughly 1,100 calories (with about 35 per cent of those coming from fat). A half pint of lager will add a further 90 calories.

### Italian

Italian food is also cereal-based – in this case either pasta or bread-dough, in the form of pizza, form the bulk of the meal. When you're eating at an Italian restaurant in England, the Fit meals to choose are those which are mostly starchy foods with low fat sauces. Tagliatelle timballo, spaghetti al pesto or ravioli con tomato e funghi will all help fill your Wheel. Avoid meats and pasta with fatty, creamy sauces (such as carbonara or marsala).

Dessert trays in Italian restaurants are a Fat trap. Ask, firmly, for fresh fruit. It will make less profit for the restaurant, but it's probably what the restaurateur eats at home in Italy.

Tagliatelle timballo with salad, followed by fresh fruit, will supply roughly 1,000 calories, and a large glass of wine will add about 140 calories.

# FEASTS

**Brain-washed by all the calorie-cutting books, slimmers believe they can never share the pleasures of a dinner party. Rubbish! On the FAT TO FIT plan, feasts are not Sin, they are In. Just keep big meals for special occasions. Earlier in the day, nibble on Fit snacks (see page 83), or try the following to bridge the gap till evening.**

### Breakfast
300 calories
Don't skip your breakfast just because you've got a feast day ahead.

### *Fruit Salad*
*100g (4oz) dried prunes*
*a sliver of lemon peel*
*1 banana, peeled and chopped*
*1 large peach, roughly chopped*

The prunes should be cooked the previous night – cover them with water in a small saucepan and simmer with the sliver of lemon for 30 minutes. Leave to soak overnight, and in the morning mix the fresh fruit with the prunes and juice. Watch out for the stones!

### Dinner Party
1,500 calories per person
All the FAT TO FIT recipes so far have been for a one-person serving. The Dinner Party recipe serves four people. You can cook the pudding and prepare the crudités in advance, then put the main dish in the oven when your guests are all assembled.

### *Crudités*
*The dip:*
*325g (12oz) chickpeas, soaked overnight*
*3 tbsp cold pressed olive oil*
*2 tbsp white wine vinegar*
*Juice of one lemon*
*3 cloves garlic, peeled and crushed*

Rinse the chickpeas and set to boil for 1½ hours, or until they are soft when pinched. Drain the chickpeas and put all the ingredients in a liquidizer. Blend at high speed until smooth. If the result looks too solid, add more vinegar and lemon.

*The vegetables:*
*225g (8oz) carrots, scrubbed*
*100g (4oz) beetroot, scrubbed*
*100g (4oz) pepper, washed and dried*
*100g (4oz) fresh tomatoes*
*100g (4oz) cucumber*
*100g (4oz) celery, washed and dried*
*100g (4oz) black olives*

Cut the carrot, pepper and celery into long, stick-like strips. Quarter the tomatoes and cut the beetroot into circular shapes. Arrange an assortment of each on four plates, with the bean dip in the middle.

### Main course: Poached Trout
*1 salmon trout (approximately 700g/1½lb) cleaned and gutted*
*Lemon juice*
*1 tbsp fresh chives*
*700g (1½lb) scrubbed new potatoes*
*350g (12oz) broccoli, washed*
*100g (4oz) almonds*

Heat the oven to gas mark 5, 185°C (370°F). Sprinkle the lemon juice, most of the chives and some black pepper into the stomach cavity of the fish and wrap it loosely in foil. Place in the oven for 20 minutes. Set the potatoes to cook at the same time. Allow about 10 minutes for the broccoli to steam thoroughly. Toast the almonds under the grill. The trout is cooked when the eyes have turned white. Serve it by running a sharp knife under the backbone and dividing each fillet into two. Garnish the fish with the chives and scatter almonds on the broccoli.

### Pudding: Pears au Cointreau
*450g (1lb) pears*
*400ml (¾ pint) orange juice*
*8ml (3fl oz) Cointreau*
*225g (8oz) plain yoghurt*

Place the pears and orange juice in a saucepan, bring to the boil and simmer for 30 minutes, or until pears are soft. Then add the Cointreau, and either serve hot or cold, passing round the yoghurt separately.

### Drink:
*2 glasses (approximately 100ml/3½fl oz each) white wine*
*2 cups of coffee with skimmed milk*

# PACKED LUNCH AND PICNICS

You're already wise to the difference between Fat and Fit snacks. The guide is on page 83. Here's how to prepare Fit packed lunches (and see page 23). Or how about a long weekend walk and a picnic?

## Packed Lunch
700 calories
Making your own packed lunch is an excellent way of ensuring you get a Fit midday meal.

> 4 slices of wholemeal bread (50g/2oz each approximately)
> 50g (2oz) tuna, drained of oil and flaked
> ½ a large banana
> 1 carton plain yoghurt (160g/6oz approximately)
> 1 apple, 1 large orange (or fruit to taste)

Make one tuna and one banana sandwich, wrap and put in a box with the yoghurt (don't forget a spoon!), apple and orange.

## Picnic Lunch
700 calories
Here's a picnic lunch to take on your long walk.

> 100g (4oz) chicken on bone, baked and skinned
> 175g (6oz) new potatoes, washed, scrubbed and boiled in their skins
> fresh mint and chives, chopped
> 1 tbsp plain yoghurt
> 50g (2oz) courgette, steamed, washed and sliced
> 100g (4oz) endive, washed and shredded
> 25g (1oz) cashew nuts
> 1 quarter lemon
> ½ small melon or ¼ a large one
> 1 wholemeal roll

Wrap up the chicken in foil. Dice the potatoes and mix together with the mint, chives and yoghurt. Place in a journey-proof container. Mix the courgette, endive and cashew nuts together in another container. Pack the roll, melon and lemon slice. When you are ready to eat, sprinkle the salad with fresh lemon juice. Enjoy yourself!

These Fit meals for a week were devised by Adriana Luba, Deirdre McQuillan and Felicity Lawrence. Text by Geoffrey Cannon, Deirdre McQuillan and Felicity Lawrence. Nutritional analyses here and throughout the book by Adriana Luba, and Wendy Doyle of the Nuffield Laboratories, London.

# FAT TO FIT

## 10

# THE ACTION PLAN

**A**t home, at work, outdoors; weekdays, weekends, holidays: now you know that it's all about recovering your lost energy, with everyday activity. But how do you do it? ● Here is your plan of action, to use at work and at home, to suit you and your own style of life ● What if you are chained to a desk? What if you have small children? Here are some answers ● And here, too, are some ideas on how to take it further. Remember, more action in the fresh air means that you'll be fitter for more whole food

The charts on the next four pages are designed to encourage you to find your own way to fitness.

If you have a desk job there's not a lot you can do to make the job itself much more active. You can walk around more and use the stairs, true. But as the charts show, a good plan is to restore an extra 100 calories to your journey to and from work; gain another 100 at work (including the lunch hour); and get up to a total of an extra 300 a day with another 100 at home.

Part of the skill in moving from Fat to Fit at home is noticing when you quite fancy doing something by hand rather than by machine. Most of all enjoy walking – to the shops, to appointments, for pleasure.

# FAT DAY AT WORK

An average woman nowadays is in energy balance, neither losing nor gaining fat, at 2000 calories, of which about one calorie a minute (1440 a day) is for the body's own workings (Basal Metabolic Rate or BMR) and another 200 for digestion (Specific Dynamic Action or SDA). A mere 360 or so is for other activity. Here is a diary of one Fat day at work.

| Time (hr/min) | Activity (calories) | Calories (minute)* | Calories (total)* |
|---|---|---|---|
| **0.30** | **Getting up: 13** | | |
| 0.10 | Washing | 0.5 | 5 |
| 0.10 | Dressing | 0.5 | 5 |
| 0.10 | Eating | 0.3 | 3 |
| **1.30** | **Travelling: 67** | | |
| 1.15 | Car/bus/train (average) | 0.5 | 37 |
| 0.15 | Walking slowly | 2.0 | 30 |
| **7.00** | **At work: 176** | | |
| 6.40 | Sedentary desk-type work (average) | 0.3 | 120 |
| 0.20 | Walking slowly | 2.0 | 40 |
| **1.00** | **Lunchtime** | | |
| 0.20 | Eating | 0.3 | 6 |
| 0.40 | Sitting and talking | 0.25 | 10 |
| **6.00** | **At home: 104** | | |
| 0.20 | Cooking | 1.5 | 30 |
| 0.15 | Eating | 0.3 | 5 |
| 0.30 | Housework (light): tidying, making beds, washing up, dusting, mending (average) | 1.0 | 30 |
| 4.30 | Watching TV/reading | 0.1 | 27 |
| 0.15 | Bathing | 0.5 | 7 |
| 0.10 | Undressing | 0.5 | 5 |
| **16.00** | **Total activity** | | **360** |
| **24.00** | Basal Metabolic Rate incl. 8 hours sleep | | 1440 |
| | Specific Dynamic Action (digestion) | | 200 |
| | **Total calories** | | **2000** |

Men: add 30 per cent to all figures                    *additional to BMR

# FIT DAY AT WORK

Here's how you can plan to recover 300 calories a day of activity if you have a desk job. This diary shows an extra 100 calories used in the day's journeys; another extra 100 at work; and the final 100, making 300 extra calories in all, after work. Figures are additional to BMR, SDA, and to the 360 calories of activity used in the Fat day opposite.

| Time (hr/min) | Activity (calories) | Calories (minute)* | Calories (total)* |
|---|---|---|---|
| 0.30 | **Getting up: 13** | 0.3–0.5 | 13 |
| **1.30** | **Travelling: 167** | | |
| 0.55 | Car/bus/train (average) | 0.5 | 27 |
| 0.35 | Walking fast/cycling | 4.0 | 140 |
| **7.00** | **At work: 276** | | |
| 6.20 | Sedentary desk-type work | 0.3 | 114 |
| 0.35 | Walking a little faster | 2.25 | 79 |
| 0.05 | Climbing stairs | 6.0 | 30 |
| **1.00** | **Lunchtime** | | |
| 0.20 | Eating | 0.3 | 6 |
| 0.25 | Sitting and talking | 0.25 | 6 |
| 0.15 | Walking briskly | 2.75 | 41 |
| **6.00** | **At home: 204** | | |
| 0.20 | Cooking | 1.5 | 30 |
| 0.30 | Eating | 0.3 | 9 |
| 0.20 | Housework (light) | 1.0 | 20 |
| 0.15 | Housework (heavier): cleaning, polishing, gardening etc. (average) | 2.0 | 30 |
| 0.20 | Walking briskly/recreation | 2.75 | 55 |
| 3.50 | Watching TV/reading | 0.2 | 48 |
| 0.15 | Bathing | 0.5 | 7 |
| 0.10 | Undressing Love-making** | 0.5 | 5 |
| **16.00** | **Total Activity** | | **660** |
| **24.00** | Basal Metabolic Rate incl. 8 hours sleep | | 1440 |
| | Specific Dynamic Action (digestion) | | 200 |
| | **Total calories** | | **2300** |

Men: add 30 per cent to all figures    * additional to BMR
** bonus for Fit people

# FAT DAY AT HOME

Cars, central heating, TV and domestic machines mean that a mother at home may gain fat if she eats more than 2000 calories a day. Here is a diary of one Fat day at home. Notice that walking is almost eliminated from the daily routine, and cooking, along with ten minutes' play with the children is the only active part of the day. Is this you?

| Time (hr/min) | Activity (calories) | Calories (minute)* | Calories (total)* |
|---|---|---|---|
| **1.30** | **Getting up: 39** | | |
| 0.30 | Washing incl. children | 0.5 | 15 |
| 0.30 | Dressing incl. children | 0.5 | 15 |
| 0.30 | Eating incl. with children | 0.3 | 9 |
| **0.30** | **Travelling (school): 15** | | |
| 0.30 | Car/bus (average) | 0.5 | 15 |
| **6.00** | **At home (day): 156** | | |
| 1.00 | Housework (light) (average) | 1.0 | 60 |
| 1.00 | Shopping (little walking) (average) | 0.5 | 30 |
| 0.20 | Cook lunch | 1.5 | 30 |
| 0.20 | Eating | 0.3 | 6 |
| 1.40 | Watching TV/reading | 0.1 | 10 |
| 1.40 | Talking, telephoning | 0.2 | 20 |
| **8.00** | **At home (evening): 150** | | |
| 0.20 | Cooking | 1.5 | 30 |
| 0.30 | Eating incl. with children | 0.3 | 9 |
| 0.10 | Play with children | 2.2 | 22 |
| 0.20 | Housework (light) (average) | 1.0 | 20 |
| 1.20 | Talking | 0.2 | 16 |
| 4.30 | Watching TV/reading | 0.1 | 27 |
| 0.25 | Bathing incl. children | 0.5 | 13 |
| 0.25 | Undress incl. children | 0.5 | 13 |
| **16.00** | **Total activity** | | **360** |
| **24.00** | Basal Metabolic Rate incl. 8 hours sleep | | 1440 |
| | Specific Dynamic Action (digestion) | | 200 |
| | **Total calories** | | **2000** |

Men: add 30 per cent to all figures          *additional to BMR

# FIT DAY AT HOME

If you have children it's fun being Fit. This diary shows an extra 100 calories used with your kids before and after school; another extra 100 in the house; and the third extra 100 at play, with your family. If you don't have children, go for walks anyway and be active in the evenings. Exercise – dancing, jogging, swimming – uses calories up faster.

| Time (hr/min) | Activity (calories) | Calories (minute)* | Calories (total)* |
|---|---|---|---|
| **1.55** | **Getting up: 94** | | |
| 1.30 | Washing, dressing, eating | 0.3–0.5 | 39 |
| 0.25 | Play with children | 2.2 | 55 |
| **0.30** | **Travelling (school): 60** | | |
| 0.30 | Walking slowly | 2.0 | 60 |
| **5.35** | **At home (day): 256** | | |
| 1.00 | Housework (light) (av) | 1.0 | 60 |
| 1.00 | Shopping (some walking) | 2.0 | 120 |
| 0.20 | Cook lunch | 1.5 | 30 |
| 0.20 | Eating | 0.3 | 6 |
| 0.25 | Writing/sewing/drawing | 0.6 | 15 |
| 0.50 | Watching TV/reading | 0.1 | 5 |
| 1.40 | Talking/telephoning | 0.2 | 20 |
| **8.00** | **At home (evening): 250** | | |
| 0.20 | Cooking | 1.5 | 30 |
| 0.30 | Eating incl. with children | 0.3 | 9 |
| 0.25 | Play with children | 2.2 | 55 |
| 0.20 | Housework (light) | 1.0 | 20 |
| 0.10 | Housework (heavier) | 2.0 | 20 |
| 0.10 | Walking briskly/recreation | 2.75 | 28 |
| 1.45 | Talking | 0.2 | 21 |
| 3.30 | TV/reading/standing | 0.2 | 42 |
| 0.50 | Bathing, undress | 0.5 | 25 |
| | Love-making** | | |
| **16.00** | **Total activity** | | **660** |
| **24.00** | Basal Metabolic Rate incl. 8 hours sleep | | 1440 |
| | Specific Dynamic Action (digestion) | | 200 |
| | **Total calories** | | **2300** |

Men: add 30 percent to all figures     * additional to BMR
** bonus for Fit people

Looking at the charts in this chapter, you may feel that the 'Diaries' outlined don't apply to you. One shows the move from Fat to Fit for a woman with an office job and no children who, as you will have noticed, shops so casually that 'shopping' doesn't even appear in her day's activities. The others show Fat and Fit days for a mother at home.

Men use round about thirty per cent more energy. If you are a man you can use the tables without needing a calculator: just make the swaps from Fat inactivity to Fit activity that suit you. And both men and women can pick up more ideas from the charts on pages 61 and 134.

You may feel that you are far more active than shown in the Fat 'diaries'. There are plenty of people who are liable to gain fat, yet who are a lot more active than shown in the two Fat days. There's no need to use the Fat days at work or at home as a base. Simply work out your own way of adding 300 more calories of activity every day to your own life (400 if you are a man). And after three months or so, measure your waistline and check out how you feel.

Energy breeds energy. Remember that the human body is a machine that improves with use, and that we are designed for action. The plan of FAT TO FIT is that you find your own way to become twice as active as (say) your neighbour or the person at the next desk.

What about sport, and formal exercise? Don't run before you can walk. But when you are ready to run, or swim, or dance, then you'll become more and more energetic, and that means, in turn, that you can enjoy more food. It's now four o'clock on a freezing February afternoon, and I'm finishing this chapter. Carl Gardner, FAT TO FIT editor, and I are about to go on our daily run round Hyde Park. It takes forty minutes, we both weigh twelve stone, and we'll use up an extra 560 calories. Carl has worked out that his run is worth almost a bottle of white wine. Over a week my daily run is worth a pound of body fat. And that's not counting the extra value of sustained vigorous exercise. Cheers! Good health!●

# FAT TO FIT

## 11

# THE WHEEL REVEALED

**T**he Wheel of Health, used throughout this book, works as a map of nourishment. It shows at a glance the value of the food we eat. It can be used to reveal the value of a single item of food, a meal, and of the food supply of a nation ● Presented for the first time in book form, the Wheel brings together the very latest scientific knowledge and judgement on food and health in a way that anybody can use ● How does the Wheel work? What principles is it based on? And why is it the most reliable guide yet devised to your food and your health? Here, for the reader with a special interest, is the Wheel revealed

How good, or how bad, is the quality of the food produced and eaten in Britain? Much highly processed food manufactured in this country is drained or empty of nourishment and much of it (saturated fats and processed sugars notably), is harmful to health in the quantities typically consumed. The very last thing that a basically sedentary population should eat is food supplying calories without nourishment.

It is, though, possible to answer the question more precisely. For health and life itself, we cannot do without essential nutrients; they are not made within the body, so we have to eat them, as food. What are these essential nutrients? What amount do we need for health? And what amount do we actually consume? All this information is available, but until now has not been all assembled together.

The Wheel of Health, shown here, is designed to be a map of nourishment (or in scientific language, 'nutrient density'). It can be used to show the quality of one particular food or a whole meal; or the quality of the diet eaten by an individual man, woman or child; or a group within the population; or – as here – a nation. Every Wheel is scaled to represent a given amount of calories. Thus a breakfast Wheel is for a meal of 400 calories, a lunch Wheel for 700 calories and so on.

The nutrients are represented on the twenty-eight segments of the Wheel. The four large segments at the top of the Wheel show proteins, starches, fibres and essential fats. The bottom half of the Wheel shows twelve vitamins (left) and twelve minerals (right). When a segment is full – shaded in from the centre to the circumference – this illustrates food supplying enough, or more than enough, of that particular nutrient for the given amount of energy. A full Wheel shows a fully balanced meal – or diet.

All the nutrients recommended for good health[1] are scaled so that the recommended amount (or in some cases the mid-point of 'a safe and adequate range') is on the circumference of the Wheel. Being a picture of health, the Wheel does not show processed sugars or saturated fats, which are not essential and potentially harmful; nor monounsaturated fats, believed to be harmless but also not essential.

The sources of information for the Wheel are as follows. For the amount of essential nutrients in the national diet, for the most part data from the Ministry of Agriculture, Fisheries and Food (MAFF) is used, either from the most recent annual report of the National Food Survey,[2] or else

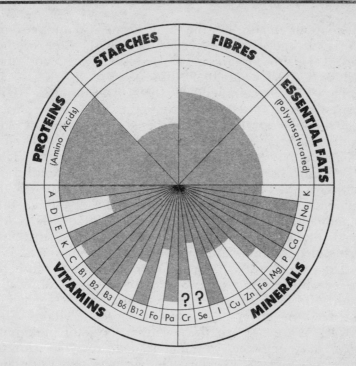

● **Fat Wheel: The British national food supply.** This Wheel (also printed on the back cover and on page 97) shows that the average supply of food has enough proteins and the more familiar vitamins. But it is sadly deficient in starches, fibres, essential fats, some minerals and vitamins D, E and the B complex group. Poorer sections of the population may have a much greater shortfall of essential nutrients.

from occasional papers, published at different times in a variety of scientific journals, by MAFF staff.[3-11] In a couple of cases, finding no British source, American data[12, 13] is used.

The recommendations for the amount of nutrients needed are: those published in 1980, and confirmed in 1985, by the National Academy of Sciences in the USA[1] (proteins, vitamins, minerals) together with other recommendations made by the US Senate Committee on Nutrition and Human Needs[14] (starches), those of the World Health Organisation[15] (essential fats), and the British NACNE committee[16] (fibres).

The UK Recommended Dietary Allowances (UK RDAs)[17] are not used here because they are not much use. The thinking on which they are based is half a century old, dating back beyond 1945 when the Ministry of Food's *Manual of Nutrition*[18] was first published. Since then UK RDAs have been changed little and are for a handful of nutrients only: protein (an RDA higher than in the USA); vitamins A, D, calcium, iron (lower); $B_1$, $B_2$, $B_3$ (much the same); and C (half that of the US RDA). If UK RDAs are used, the British diet is adequate or marginal in these 'scheduled' vitamins and minerals; and high in protein.

The American recommendations (US RDAs) used here are sometimes criticized in Britain for being unrealistically high. This is because they are goals not readily reached if the diet is mostly made up of highly processed foods. The UK RDAs are based on the negative concept of 'minimum plus', meaning the amount needed to avoid clinical deficiency diseases, like scurvy or beri-beri, plus a substantial safety margin. The US RDAs are based, where possible, on the concept of 'tissue saturation', which suggests an amount needed for positive health and protection against disease. The American recommendations are therefore used here.[19]

As an example, then, it can be seen from the Wheel on page 183 that the UK average national food supply is adequate in vitamins A, C (almost), $B_1$, $B_2$ and $B_3$. This is not altogether surprising: manufacturers are encouraged to add these vitamins to processed food.[20] However, the national food supply is short of the fat-soluble vitamins D and E, and vitamins in the water-soluble B complex ($B_6$ and folic acid, shown as Fo). These vitamins have a vast number of functions. For instance, D (also supplied through sunlight) protects against weakening of the bones,[1,17] E (probably) against cancers,[21,22] folic acid (almost certainly) against birth defects.[23,24] These conditions are common in Britain.

Minerals (the twelve small segments to the right of vitamins) may be inert, or, like lead, toxic. The twelve represented on the Wheel are all essential nutrients. So it can be seen that the UK average national food supply is adequate in calcium (Ca) and iodine (I). Again this is not surprising; as with the 'scheduled' vitamins mentioned above, shortage of these minerals was officially recognised as a public health problem half a century ago[18] and steps taken to solve the problem. Calcium, for example, is still added to white flour and thus to white bread, in the form of chalk.[25] However, despite iron (Fe) also being scheduled, many people and most women of child-bearing age are short of it.

The picture shown by the Wheel of Health underestimates, in an important respect, the public health problem represented by the British national food supply. This is because the Wheel shows the 'average' diet. By definition, half of any population is worse off than the average. The Ministry of Agriculture only releases a small amount of the data available on sections of the population consuming less than average amounts of nutrients[2]. But this, and international comparison with figures available for the USA and European countries,[26] strongly suggests that the worse-off ten or twenty-five per cent of the British population consume inadequate amounts of a large number of essential nutrients●

# REFERENCES

1. National Research Council. *Recommended dietary allowances*, ninth revised edition. (Washington: National Academy of Sciences, 1980).

2. Ministry of Agriculture, Fisheries and Food. *Household food consumption and expenditure: 1984.* (London: HMSO, 1986).

3. Wenlock R., Buss D. 'New estimates of fibre in the British diet'. *British Medical Journal*, 1984; 288; 1873.

4. Bull N., Buss D. 'Biotin, pantothenic acid and vitamin E in the British household food supply'. *Human Nutrition: Applied Nutrition*, 1982; 36A: 190–196.

5. Spring J., Robertson J., Buss D. 'Trace nutrients. 3: Magnesium, copper, zinc,

vitamin B6, vitamin B12 and folic acid in the British household food supply'. *British Journal of Nutrition,* 1979; 41: 487–493.

6. Poh Tan S., Wenlock R., Buss D. 'Folic acid content of the diet in various types of British household'. *Human Nutrition: Applied Nutrition,* 1984; 38A: 17–22.

7. Bull N., Buss D. 'Contributions of food to potassium intakes'. *Proceedings of the Nutrition Society,* 1980; 39: 30A.

8. Bull N., Buss D. 'Contributions of food to sodium intakes'. *Proceedings of the Nutrition Society,* 1980; 39: 30A.

9. Wenlock R., Buss D. 'Trace nutrients. 4: iodine in British food'. *British Journal of Nutrition,* 1982; 47: 381–390.

10. Thorn J., Robertson J., Buss D. 'Trace nutrients. Selenium in British food'. *British Journal of Nutrition,* 1978; 39: 391–396.

11. Buss D. 'Essential trace nutrients in the UK diet'. *Chemistry and Industry,* 4 July 1983.

12. Olson R. 'Vitamin K'. *Modern Nutrition in Health and Disease,* ed. Goodhart R. *et al.* (Philadelphia: Lee and Febiger, 1973).

13. Kumpulainen J., Wolf C., Veillon C., Mertz W. 'Determination of chromium in selected United States diets'. *Journal of Agriculture and Food Chemistry,* 1979; 27: 490–494.

14. Select Committee on Nutrition and Human Needs. *Dietary goals for the United States.* (Washington: US Government Printing Office, 1977).

15. World Health Organisation. *Prevention of coronary heart disease.* (General: WHO, 1982).

16. National Advisory Committee on Nutrition Education. *A discussion paper on proposals for nutritional guidelines for health education in Britain.* (London: Health Education Council, 1983).

17. Department of Health and Social Security: Committee on Medical Aspects of Food Policy. *Recommended intakes of nutrients in the United Kingdom.* (London: HMSO, 1969, 1979, 1981).

18. *Manual of Nutrition.* (London: HMSO, 1945, 1953).

19. Levels on the Wheels are either the US RDAs or else the mid-point of the 'safe and adequate range'. These are as follows for vitamins: Vitamin A, 1mg; D, 5mcg; E, 10mg; K, 105mcg; C, 60mg; $B_1$, 1.5mg; $B_2$, 1.6mg; $B_3$, 18mg; $B_6$, 2.2mg; $B_{12}$, 3mcg; Folic acid (Fo), 400mcg; Pantothenic acid (Pa), 5.5mg.

For minerals, the mid-point of the 'safe and adequate range' is: K, 3750mg; Na, 2200mg; Cl, 3400mg (note, K/Na ratio of about 5 to 3); Ca, 800mg; P, 800mg; Mg, 350mg (note, Ca/P ratio of 1 to 1); Fe, 18mg; Zn, 15mg; Cu, 3mg (note, Fe/Zn/Cu ratio of about 6 to 6 to 1); I, 150mcg; Se, 125mcg; Cr, 125mcg.

20. *Statutory instruments: The food labelling regulations 1984.* (London: HMSO, 1984).

21. National Research Council: Committee on Diet, Nutrition and Cancer. *Diet, Nutrition and Cancer.* (Washington; National Academy Press, 1982).

22. Willett W., MacMahon B. 'Diet and cancer: an overview'. *New England Journal of Medicine,* 1984; 310: 633–638, 697–703.

23. Smithells R. *et al.* 'Further evidence of vitamin supplementation for prevention of neural tube defect recurrences'. *Lancet,* 1983; I: 1027–1031.

24. Smithells R. 'Prevention of neural tube defects by vitamin supplementation' in *Prevention of Spina Bifida and other Neural Tube Defects,* ed Dobbing J. (London: Academic Press, 1983).

25. Department of Health and Social Security: Committee on medical aspects of food policy. *Nutritional aspects of bread and flour.* (London: HMSO, 1981).

26. Wynn M., Wynn A. Personal communication.

# FAT TO FIT

## 12

# FROM FIT TO SUPERFIT

**So now you know how to fill your Wheel of Health and how to put back that lost activity into your everyday life. Gradually, over six months maybe, or a year, you'll progress from Fat to Fit. You may lose a lot of weight, or you may not; but you'll be slimmer ● So, once you've got rid of that extra fat, what then? FAT TO FIT isn't a tedious regime, to be abandoned and forgotten: it really is the healthy way of life ● Can you go further? The answer is yes. Once you and your family have become accustomed to enjoying good food and once you really are thriving on all that extra activity, you can use FAT TO FIT as the foundation for a new Superfit life**

Give it time and FAT TO FIT will work for every able-bodied person who wants to lose ten or even thirty pounds of excess fat. And nourishing food, together with regular activity, is the only sound foundation for fat loss if you are very overweight. What's next, once you really are fit, eating your fill of good food and enjoying plenty of every-day activity?

The Wheel of Health on page 188 is the Superfit wheel, busting out all over with nourishment. The point is that

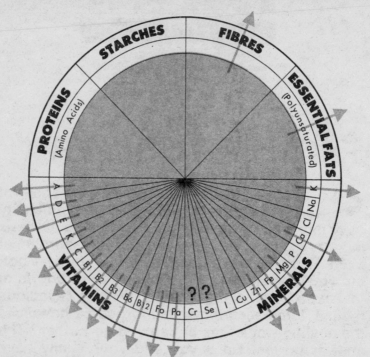

● **Superfit Wheel of Health.** Two hours a week of really vigorous exercise will take you most of the way from Fit to Superfit; and you'll have room for lots of whole fresh food. Superfit people can eat as much as they like without putting on fat. A Superfit Wheel is super-rich in fibres, essential fats, all the vitamins and some minerals. For proteins and other minerals and trace elements, you can have too much of a good thing.

the more active you are, the more food you can enjoy; and the more food you eat, the more nourishment your body will get. An 'average' woman is in energy balance at around 2,000 calories a day – the figure for men is around 2,600 calories a day.

Once you have found your lost 300–400 calories a day of activity and put it back into your life, you will be above the top end of the 'average' energy balance range.

# TAKING IT FURTHER

This training schedule, building up to two hours a week of vigorous exercise, will take you from Fit to Superfit. Take each stage at your own pace. Remember that it has taken years for your body to get out of shape; it will take a number of months to regain the pleasure in exercise that most children enjoy. As a rough guide, most people I have worked with take around ten to twenty weeks to reach stage 5.

It's important to base an exercise on the 'one day on, one day off' principle. Give your body time to rebuild and become stronger on the day after exercise. Build up to a four-day-a-week schedule gradually. The days shown here for exercise assume that it suits you to take extra time out during the weekend. If not, devise a schedule to suit yourself.

You can of course 'mix' different types of exercise, if you like the idea of going running one day, swimming another, and dancing on a third day.

## THE SEVEN STAGES AND THE 49 STEPS

|         | Sat. | Sun. | Mon. | Tues. | Wed. | Thurs. | Fri. | Total |
|---------|------|------|------|-------|------|--------|------|-------|
| Stage 1 | 10   | —    | —    | 5     | —    | 5      | —    | 20    |
| Stage 2 | 15   | —    | —    | 5     | —    | 10     | —    | 30    |
| Stage 3 | 20   | —    | —    | 10    | —    | 10     | —    | 40    |
| Stage 4 | 25   | 10   | —    | 10    | —    | 15     | —    | 60    |
| Stage 5 | 30   | 15   | —    | 15    | —    | 20     | —    | 80    |
| Stage 6 | 35   | 15   | —    | 25    | —    | 25     | —    | 100   |
| Stage 7 | 40   | 20   | —    | 30    | —    | 30     | —    | 120   |

Figures are in minutes per exercise session.

If you choose to build not just regular activity, but also vigorous exercise, into your everyday life, your energy balance will continue to rise. Look at the exercise schedule on this page, adapted from *Dieting Makes You Fat*. This is a plan for a steady build-up from twenty minutes to two hours a week of running, dancing, swimming, 'aerobics', gym work or other really vigorous exercise.

You don't have to be a fanatic to move from Fit to

Superfit. It's really a question of re-gaining the joy in everyday exercise that healthy children and animals have naturally. Recently, while running round Hyde Park in central London, I saw two examples of Superfit people. One was running with her dog. The other was a father of two daughters who were aged maybe ten and fourteen – all were running together.

Running is the exercise of my choice. Dancing or 'aerobics' is just as good. For the fit person who still has excess fat to budge, the beauty of steady, vigorous exercise, sustained for at least thirty minutes at a time, is that it speeds up your overall metabolic rate. You feel warmer all the time and, yes, this means you can eat more and more delicious food and yet get leaner, too.

As you will have seen, the food you can make to fill your Wheel of Health is all readily found at any well-stocked supermarket. You don't have to be a food fanatic, either, to gain health and fitness. But yes, you can go further. For example, food loses nourishment when it is cooked, so vegetables are best cooked lightly. At the same time, raw vegetables are even more nourishing.

The best way to move from Fit to Superfit food, so that your Wheel of Health really does bust out all over, is to do what people all over the world have done for many thousands of years: eat lots and lots of high-quality, wholegrain cereal and masses of vegetables, pulses, legumes and fruit; use high-quality oils; and eat meat and sweet things just as relishes, together with herbs and spices.

The fact is that anybody who knows about good food, and cares a lot about it, will not enjoy the food served up in most restaurants, nor much of the food offered by friends. Superfit people are picky and choosy. Much depends, of course, on how much trouble you want to take with your life●

# FAT TO FIT

# ADDITIVES TO ZINC

**N**ow we know that responsibility for our own health and fitness is largely in our own hands. Food, health and fitness have suddenly become subjects of intense interest. And most people in Britain, America and other Western countries want to get rid of excess fat ● But what do all the words mean? Special sections throughout FAT TO FIT have defined the key ideas. This section, part index, part little dictionary, tells you all you need to know ● Finally there's a further reading list, and a key to the terms used on the 'menus' and Wheels of Health

**additives** are what living in a modern society is all about, say the food manufacturers. Additives, says the CIA (Chemical Industries Association) preserve food and protect us from all keeling over from food poisoning. But less (by weight, volume of value) than one hundredth of food additives are preservatives. The main function of additives is to tart up cheap and nasty ingredients – like saturated fats, processed starches and sugars, and salt – to make them look, smell, taste and feel like good food. Most highly processed food sold nowadays is contaminated and/or adulterated with additives. *See* **FACT**.

**bacon.** Fat food.     **22, 148**

**Bacon and Meat**     **93**
**Manufacturers Association.**
Trade association set up to
protect the interests of the
manufacturers in
Westminster, Whitehall and
Brussels.

**balance.** What everybody     **74, 90,**
needs for good health, is a     **181**
balanced diet. That's what
all the books say. But what
is a 'balanced diet'? That's
what the Wheel of Health
is all about. A full Wheel
shows food supplying all
the vital nutrients you
need, in the right
proportion. In Britain the
official 'balanced' diet is
based on the science of half
a century ago, and ignores
most nutrients now known
to be vital for fitness and
health.

**basal metabolic rate (BMR)**     **60, 77**
**Beeton, Mrs**     **112**
**Beverly Hills diet**     **95–96**
**biscuits.** Fat food.     **146, 148**
**bread.** Eat lots of bread,     **26–28**
but only good quality
wholemeal.

**breakfast.** Chapter 2.     **33**

**British Nutrition**     **89**
**Foundation (BNF).** Food
industry-funded
association of experts,
originally set up as a forum
for the best information
about food and health.
Said by some to be over-
protective of industry.

**brunch.** Chapter 6     **105**
**bulimia**     **95**
**Burkitt, Dr Denis**     **56**
**butter.** Fat food.     **146, 148**

**Butter Information Council**     **93**
**(BIC).** Trade association
set up to protect the

interests of the
manufacturers, in
Westminster, Whitehall
and Brussels.

**cake.** Processed cakes are     **146, 148**
Fat food. Home-made
scones and fruit cake are
fine for a treat.

**Cake and Biscuit Alliance**     **93**
**(CBA).** Trade association
set up to protect the
interests of the
manufacturers, in
Westminster, Whitehall,
and Brussels. Known as the
Sweet Fat Alliance or Sweet
FA for short.

**calcium (Ca)**     **90**
**calorie.** A unit of energy.     **47, 60–64**
For a woman, average
daily requirement of
calories is around 2,000 a
day, which is what the FAT
TO FIT plans are based
on. Advertisements for
processed food often seem
to suggest that the
products supply lots of
energy but are low in
calories. Piffle! The word
'calorie' is short for
kiloCalorie, sometimes
shown as kCal.

**calorie-cutting diets**     **94**
**cancer**     **75, 128, 185**
**carbohydrates**     **40, 42**
**cardiovascular system**     **59**
**cellulose**     **42, 59**
**cereal.** Wholegrain cereal     **33–44**
is the staff of life.

**cereals.** Ready-to-eat     **33–44**
breakfast cereals are often
loaded with sugars and
salt. Look at the label.

**cheese.** Fat food, mostly.     **25, 146, 148**
Stick to small portions of
mature cheeses.

**chemicals.** *See* **additives.**

your doctor is no help, try contacting your local community dietitian.

**eggs.** OK once in a while.    146, 148
**energy.** Everybody needs    60
energy. But people in Western countries use a lot less personal energy than in the days before the car and central heating. As a result Western people are in artificially low energy balance, and find it hard to get enough nourishment from food without consuming too much energy (calories) for their sedentary bodies' needs. The answer to this problem of modern society? FAT TO FIT.

**FACT.** Food Additives Campaign Team. An association of representative groups, set up in December 1985, to demand a more responsible use of food additives. Supported by MPs of all parties.
**fast food.** Often Fat food.    81–88, 132
**fat,** meaning fats in food,    114, 132
is the word that strikes horror into the heart of every slimmer. With some reason, too, because all fats are heavy in calories (energy). And with further reason in the case of saturated fats, a prime cause of heart disease. However, 'fat' is an out-of-date word. The proper word is 'fats'. This is because some fats are bad for you: these are saturated fats (SFAs), trans fatty acids, hydrogenated fats, and any other hard or hardened fats. Cut them right out. The good news is that other fats are positively good for your health: these are essential fats (EFAs), polyunsaturated fats (PUFAs), and specific essential fats, notably linoleic acid and eicosapentaenoic acid (EPA). While these are, like all fats, heavy in calories, everybody, including slimmers, should consume them in whole, fresh food such as wholegrain cereal, oily fish, nuts and seeds.

**fat farms**    94
**feasting.** Big meals are    121–134, 172
Sin. That's what every calorie-cutting diet book says. So anybody who believes the diet books, and who wants to lose excess fat, says goodbye to the special pleasures of feasts, which throughout history have marked great occasions. But think again. Every community of people throughout history has feasted. But few people, until the last 200 years, have got fat. Once you become active, and once you reserve feasts for real feast days, magnificent meals can be part of the FAT TO FIT plan.

green vegetables, salads:
feast on them all. Eat them
raw, or cook them lightly.

work has become a dirty
word in Western societies.
We are told that we ought
to want machines to do our
work for us, so our bodies
decay and become fat from
neglect. The human body
is a machine that improves
with use.

yoghurt. Low fat is Fit
food. Full fat is fine for a
treat. 'Fruit flavour'
yoghurts are Fat food,
loaded with sugars and
chemicals.

# KEY TO THE MEALS AND THE WHEELS

There are 'menus' for the Fat meals and the Fit meals in this book, on pages 23, 35, 51, 67, 83, 107, 123, and 139. Below these menus are analyses showing the quality of the meals.

First, there is a band of information on the 'bad news' about the meals: their content of saturated fats, added processed sugars, salt (sodium), and chemical additives. These are marked HEAVY, MEDIUM or LIGHT. The more processed any meal, the more fats, added sugars, salt and additives it is likely to contain. Some Fit meals contain a fair amount of salt, if only because all bread is fairly salty.

The next band of information shows the 'good news' (or lack of it) about the nutrients that also supply energy or bulk to food: these are proteins, starches, fibres and essential fats. For more information about these vital nutrients, see the boxed information on pages 42–43, 58–59, 114–115 and 130–131. If a meal supplies less than two thirds of the recommended amount of the nutrient, the word used is POOR. A bit above that level – two thirds to three quarters – is POOR/MEDIUM. The next grade up, MEDIUM, means that the meal isn't a bad source of the nutrient but falls short significantly. RICH means anything between a full and a super-full segment of the wheel. Food is SUPER-RICH when it supplies more than twice the recommended amount of the nutrient.

The third and fourth bands of information at the bottom of the menus show selected vitamins and minerals, and whether the meals are POOR, POOR/MEDIUM, MEDIUM, RICH or SUPER-RICH sources of these vital nutrients. See also pages 74–75 and 90–91.

The key to the terms and abbreviations used is as follows:

| Vitamins | | Minerals and trace elements | |
|---|---|---|---|
| A | retinol equivs. or carotene | K | potassium |
| D | cholecalciferol | Na | sodium |
| E | alpha-tocopherol equivs. | Cl | chloride |
| K | | Ca | calcium |
| C | ascorbic acid | P | phosphorus |
| $B_1$ | thiamine | Mg | magnesium |
| $B_2$ | riboflavin | Fe | iron |
| $B_3$ | niacin | Zn | zinc |
| $B_6$ | pyridoxine | Cu | copper |
| $B_{12}$ | cobalamin | I | iodine |
| Fo | folic acid, or folate | Se | selenium |
| Pa | pantothenic acid | Cr | chromium |

The queries (?) against Se and Cr on all the Wheels indicate uncertainty about the levels of these trace elements in many foods.

# NOW READ ON

If you would like to know more about the ideas on which FAT TO FIT is based, or compare notes with books on the same lines, here is a short reading list. The books marked with an asterisk (*) are for the general reader. The others are more specialist, often more expensive, and probably best obtained from a good library.

Per-Olof Åstrand and Kaare Rodahl:
*Textbook of Work Physiology*
(McGraw-Hill)

Denis Burkitt:
*Don't Forget Fibre In Your Diet**
(Martin Dunitz £2.50)

Geoffrey Cannon and Hetty Einzig:
*Dieting Makes You Fat**
(Sphere £1.95)

T. L. Cleave
*The Saccharine Disease*
(John Wright; Bristol)

Michael and Sheilagh Crawford:
*What We Eat Today**
(Neville Spearman)

Felicity Lawrence (editor):
*Additives: Your Complete Survival Guide**
(Century £3.95)

William McArdle, Frank Katch, Victor Katch:
*Energy, Nutrition and Human Performance*
(Lea and Febiger; Philadelphia)

Robert McCarrison
*Nutrition and Health*

(The McCarrison Society; London)

Nathan Pritikin:
*The Pritikin Program For Diet and Exercise**
(Bantam £1.50)

Royal College of Physicians:
*Medical Aspects of Dietary Fibre*
(Pitman Medical)

Royal College of Physicians:
*Obesity*
(RCP, London)

Sports Council of Great Britain:
*Exercise, Health, Medicine**
(Sports Council £4.00)

Hugh Trowell, Denis Burkitt, Kenneth Heaton (editors):
*Fibre, Fibre-Depleted Foods and Disease*
(Academic Press)

Caroline Walker and Geoffrey Cannon:
*The Food Scandal**
(Century £3.95)

World Health Organisation:
*Habitual Physical Activity and Health*
(WHO; Copenhagen)